P9-DNO-335

M. Joanna Mellor, DSW
Patricia Brownell, PhD
Editors

Elder Abuse and Mistreatment: Policy, Practice, and Research

Elder Abuse and Mistreatment: Policy, Practice, and Research has been co-published simultaneously as *Journal of Gerontological Social Work*, Volume 46, Numbers 3/4 2006.

Pre-publication REVIEWS, COMMENTARIES, EVALUATIONS . . .

"**I**MPORTANT. . . . Rarely does a single book offer the reader the wealth of information and the multidimensional perspective of this collection. The contributors are academicians and practitioners in the variety of fields whose involvement is now understood to be vital to an effective response to a growing problem. Their contributions provide practical tools to professionals in several disciplines, and put forward concrete methodologies for screening, assessment, and intervention."

Betty F. Malks, MSW, CSW
Director, Santa Clara County Department of Aging and Adult Services, San Jose, California; North American Regional Representative, International Network for the Prevention of Elder Abuse

More Pre-publication
REVIEWS, COMMENTARIES, EVALUATIONS . . .

"AN IMPORTANT RESOURCE FOR COLLEGE AND UNIVERSITY STUDENTS in many areas of study. I applaud Pat Brownell and Joanna Mellor for pulling together a comprehensive selection of contributions that adds to our body of knowledge and deserves a place on many bookshelves. What impressed me overall was the diversity of the chapters and their subsequent value for a broad audience."

Pat Spadafora, MSW, Director
Sheridan Elder Research Centre (SERC)
Sheridan Institute of Technology and Advanced Learning
Oakville, Canada

The Haworth Press, Inc.

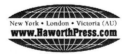

New York • London • Victoria (AU)
www.HaworthPress.com

Elder Abuse
and Mistreatment:
Policy, Practice, and Research

Elder Abuse and Mistreatment: Policy, Practice, and Research has been co-published simultaneously as *Journal of Gerontological Social Work*, Volume 46, Numbers 3/4 2006.

Elder Abuse and Mistreatment: Policy, Practice and Research, edited by M. Joanna Mellor, DSW, and Patricia Brownell, PhD (Vol. 46, No. 3/4, 2006). *"IMPORTANT. . . . Rarely does a single book offer the reader the wealth of information and the multidimensional perspective of this collection. The contributors are academicians and practitioners in the variety of fields whose involvement is now understood to be vital to an effective response to a growing problem. Their contributions provide practical tools to professionals in several disciplines, and put forward concrete methodologies for screening, assessment, and intervention." (Betty F. Malks, MSW, CSW, Director, Santa Clara County Department of Aging and Adult Services, San Jose, California; North American Regional Representative, International Network for the Prevention of Elder Abuse)*

Religion, Spirituality, and Aging: A Social Work Perspective, edited by Harry R. Moody, PhD, (Vol. 45, No. 1/2 and 3, 2005). *"From the definitive opening chapter by the eminent social gerontologist David Moberg to the erudite final chapter by Eugene Bianchi, the breadth and depth of this collection of essays provide a major contribution to the understanding of religion, spirituality, aging, and social work. These essays will both inform and challenge the reader." (Dr. Melvin A. Kimble, PhD, Professor Emeritus of Pastoral Theology and Director, Center for Aging, Religion, and Spirituality, Luther Seminary, St. Paul, Minnesota; Editor of* Viktor Frankl's Contribution to Spirituality and Aging)

Group Work and Aging: Issues in Practice, Research, and Education, edited by Robert Salmon, DSW, and Roberta Graziano, DSW (Vol. 44, No. 1/2, 2004). *Although there is a considerable amount of writing on both group work and social work with the elderly, there is surprisingly little about applying this practice method to this specific age group.* Group Work and Aging: Issues in Practice, Research, and Education *fills this gap by presenting penetrating articles about a mutual aid approach to working with diverse groups of older adults with varied needs. Respected experts and gifted researchers provide case studies, practice examples, and explanation of theory to illustrate this practice method with aging adults, their families, and their caregivers. Each well-referenced chapter delivers high quality, up-to-date social group work practice strategies to prepare practitioners for the needs of the growing population of elderly in the near future.*

Gerontological Social Work in Small Towns and Rural Communities, edited by Sandra S. Butler, PhD, and Lenard W. Kaye, DSW (Vol. 41, No. 1/2 and 3/4, 2003). *Provides a range of intervention and community skills aimed precisely at the needs of rural elders.*

Older People and Their Caregivers Across the Spectrum of Care, edited by Judith L. Howe, PhD (Vol. 40, No. 1/2, 2002). *Focuses on numerous issues relating to caregiving and social work assessment for improving quality of life for the elderly.*

Advancing Gerontological Social Work Education, edited by M. Joanna Mellor, DSW, and Joann Ivry, PhD (Vol. 39, No. 1/2, 2002). *Examines the current status of geriatric/gerontological education; offers models for curriculum development within the classroom and the practice arena.*

Gerontological Social Work Practice: Issues, Challenges, and Potential, edited by Enid Opal Cox, DSW, Elizabeth S. Kelchner, MSW, ACSW, and Rosemary Chapin, PhD, MSW (Vol. 36, No. 3/4, 2001). *This book gives you an essential overview of the role, status, and potential of gerontological social work in aging societies around the world. Drawing on the expertise of leaders in the field, it identifies key policy and practice issues and suggests directions for the future. Here you'll find important perspectives on home health care, mental health, elder abuse, older workers' issues, and death and dying, as well as an examination of the policy and practice issues of utmost concern to social workers dealing with the elderly.*

Social Work Practice with the Asian American Elderly, edited by Namkee G. Choi, PhD (Vol. 36, No. 1/2, 2001). *"Encompasses the richness of diversity among Asian Americans by including articles on Vietnamese, Japanese, Chinese, Taiwanese, Asian Indian, and Korean Americans."*

(Nancy R. Hooyman, PhD, MSW, Professor and Dean Emeritus, University of Washington School of Social Work, Seattle)

Grandparents as Carers of Children with Disabilities: Facing the Challenges, edited by Philip McCallion, PhD, ACSW, and Matthew Janicki, PhD (Vol. 33, No. 3, 2000). *Here is the first comprehensive consideration of the unique needs and experiences of grandparents caring for children with developmental disabilities. The vital information found here will assist practitioners, administrators, and policymakers to include the needs of this special population in the planning and delivery of services, and it will help grandparents in this situation to better care for themselves as well as for the children in their charge.*

Latino Elders and the Twenty-First Century: Issues and Challenges for Culturally Competent Research and Practice, edited by Melvin Delgado, PhD (Vol. 30, No. 1/2, 1998). *Explores the challenges that gerontological social work will encounter as it attempts to meet the needs of the growing number of Latino elders utilizing culturally competent principles.*

Dignity and Old Age, edited by Rose Dobrof, DSW, and Harry R. Moody, PhD (Vol. 29, No. 2/3, 1998). *"Challenges us to uphold the right to age with dignity, which is embedded in the heart and soul of every man and woman." (H. James Towey, President, Commission on Aging with Dignity, Tallahassee, FL)*

Intergenerational Approaches in Aging: Implications for Education, Policy and Practice, edited by Kevin Brabazon, MPA, and Robert Disch, MA (Vol. 28, No. 1/2/3, 1997). *"Provides a wealth of concrete examples of areas in which intergenerational perspectives and knowledge are needed." (Robert C. Atchley, PhD, Director, Scribbs Gerontology Center, Miami University)*

Social Work Response to the White House Conference on Aging: From Issues to Actions, edited by Constance Corley Saltz, PhD, LCSW (Vol. 27, No. 3, 1997). *"Provides a framework for the discussion of issues relevant to social work values and practice, including productive aging, quality of life, the psychological needs of older persons, and family issues." (Jordan I. Kosberg, PhD, Professor and PhD Program Coordinator, School of Social Work, Florida International University, North Miami, FL)*

Special Aging Populations and Systems Linkages, edited by M. Joanna Mellor, DSW (Vol. 25, No. 1/2, 1996). *"An invaluable tool for anyone working with older persons with special needs." (Irene Gutheil, DSW, Associate Professor, Graduate School of Social Service, Fordham University)*

New Developments in Home Care Services for the Elderly: Innovations in Policy, Program, and Practice, edited by Lenard W. Kaye, DSW (Vol. 24, No. 3/4, 1995). *"An excellent compilation. . . . Especially pertinent to the functions of administrators, supervisors, and case managers in home care. . . . Highly recommended for every home care agency and a must for administrators and middle managers." (Geriatric Nursing Book Review)*

Geriatric Social Work Education, edited by M. Joanna Mellor, DSW, and Renee Solomon, DSW (Vol. 18, No. 3/4, 1992). *"Serves as a foundation upon which educators and fieldwork instructors can build courses that incorporate more aging content." (SciTech Book News)*

Vision and Aging: Issues in Social Work Practice, edited by Nancy D. Weber, MSW (Vol. 17, No. 3/4, 1992). *"For those involved in vision rehabilitation programs, the book provides practical information and should stimulate readers to revise their present programs of care." (Journal of Vision Rehabilitation)*

Health Care of the Aged: Needs, Policies, and Services, edited by Abraham Monk, PhD (Vol. 15, No. 3/4, 1990). *"The chapters reflect firsthand experience and are competent and informative. Readers . . . will find the book rewarding and useful. The text is timely, appropriate, and well-presented." (Health & Social Work)*

Twenty-Five Years of the Life Review: Theoretical and Practical Considerations, edited by Robert Disch, MA (Vol. 12, No. 3/4, 1989). *This practical and thought-provoking book examines the history and concept of the life review.*

Gerontological Social Work: International Perspectives, edited by Merl C. Hokenstad, Jr., PhD, and Katherine A. Kendall, PhD (Vol. 12, No. 1/2, 1988). *"Makes a very useful contribution in examining the changing role of the social work profession in serving the elderly." (Journal of the International Federation on Ageing)*

Elder Abuse
and Mistreatment:
Policy, Practice, and Research

M. Joanna Mellor, DSW
Patricia Brownell, PhD
Editors

Elder Abuse and Mistreatment: Policy, Practice, and Research has been co-published simultaneously as *Journal of Gerontological Social Work*, Volume 46, Numbers 3/4 2006.

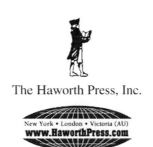

The Haworth Press, Inc.

New York • London • Victoria (AU)
www.HaworthPress.com

Elder Abuse and Mistreatment: Policy, Practice, and Research has been co-published simultaneously as *Journal of Gerontological Social Work,*[TM] Volume 46, Numbers 3/4 2006.

Cover design by Lora Wiggins

Library of Congress Catalog-in-Publication Data

Elder abuse and mistreatment : policy, practice, and research / M. Joanna Mellor, Patricia Brownell, editors.
      p. cm.
    "Co-published simultaneously as Journal of gerontological social work, Volume 46, numbers 3/4 2006."
    Includes bibliographical references and index.
    ISBN 13: 978-0-7890-3022-1 (hard cover : alk. paper)
    ISBN 10: 0-7890-3022-5 (hard cover : alk. paper)
    ISBN 13: 978-0-7890-3023-8 (soft cover : alk. paper)
    ISBN 10: 0-7890-3023-3 (soft cover : alk. paper)
    1. Older people--Abuse of. 2. Older people--Abuse of -- United States. 3. Abused elderly--Services for. 4. Abused elderly--Services for--United States. 5. Social work with older people. I. Mellor, M. Joanna. II. Brownell, Patricia J., 1943- III. Journal of gerontological social work.
  HV6626.3.E455 2006
  362.6--dc22
                                                         2006001293

Indexing, Abstracting & Website/Internet Coverage

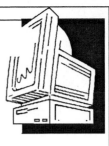

This section provides you with a list of major indexing & abstracting services and other tools for bibliographic access. That is to say, each service began covering this periodical during the year noted in the right column. Most Websites which are listed below have indicated that they will either post, disseminate, compile, archive, cite or alert their own Website users with research-based content from this work. (This list is as current as the copyright date of this publication.)

Abstracting, Website/Indexing Coverage . . . . Year When Coverage Began

- *Abstracts in Social Gerontology: Current Literature on Aging* **1989**
- *Academic Abstracts/CD-ROM* **1993**
- *Academic Search: database of 2,000 selected academic serials, updated monthly: EBSCO Publishing* **1995**
- *Academic Search Elite (EBSCO)* **1995**
- *Academic Search Premier (EBSCO) <http://www.epnet.com/ academic/acasearchprem.asp>* **1993**
- *AgeInfo CD-Rom <http://www.cpa.org.uk>* **1995**
- *AgeLine Database <http://research.aarp.org/ageline>* **1978**
- *Alzheimer's Disease Education & Referral Center (ADEAR)* **1994**
- *Applied Social Sciences Index & Abstracts (ASSIA) (Online: ASSI via Data-Star) (CDRom: ASSIA Plus) <http://www.csa.com>* **1987**
- *Behavioral Medicine Abstracts (Annals of Behavioral Medicine)* . . . **1992**
- *Biosciences Information Service of Biological Abstracts (BIOSIS), a centralized source of life science information <http://www.biosis.org>* **1993**
- *Business Source Corporate: coverage of nearly 3,350 quality magazines and journals; designed to meet the diverse information needs of corporations; EBSCO Publishing <http://www.epnet.com/ corporate/bsourcecorp.asp>* **1993**

(continued)

(continued)

(continued)

Special Bibliographic Notes related to special journal issues (separates) and indexing/abstracting:

- indexing/abstracting services in this list will also cover material in any "separate" that is co-published simultaneously with Haworth's special thematic journal issue or DocuSerial. Indexing/abstracting usually covers material at the article/chapter level.
- monographic co-editions are intended for either non-subscribers or libraries which intend to purchase a second copy for their circulating collections.
- monographic co-editions are reported to all jobbers/wholesalers/approval plans. The source journal is listed as the "series" to assist the prevention of duplicate purchasing in the same manner utilized for books-in-series.
- to facilitate user/access services all indexing/abstracting services are encouraged to utilize the co-indexing entry note indicated at the bottom of the first page of each article/chapter/contribution.
- this is intended to assist a library user of any reference tool (whether print, electronic, online, or CD-ROM) to locate the monographic version if the library has purchased this version but not a subscription to the source journal.
- individual articles/chapters in any Haworth publication are also available through the Haworth Document Delivery Service (HDDS).

Elder Abuse and Mistreatment: Policy, Practice, and Research

CONTENTS

RESEARCH

ABOUT THE EDITORS

M. Joanna Mellor, DSW, is Assistant Professor, Wurzweiler School of Social Work, Yeshiva University. Former Positions included Vice President for Information Services, Lighthouse International; Assistant Professor in the Department of Geriatrics and Adult Development, Mount Sinai Medical Center; and Executive Director of the Hunter/Mount Sinai Geriatric Education Center, a federally funded program providing geriatric education to health care professionals. Dr. Mellor has been an Adjunct Instructor at the Hunter School of Social Work since 1984 and is co-editor of *Advancing Gerontological Social Work Education, Gerontological Social Work Practice in the Community, Gerontological Social Work Practice in Long Term Care,* and the *Journal of Gerontological Social Work,* and editor of *Special Aging Populations and Systems Linkages,* all published by The Haworth Press, Inc.

Patricia Brownell, PhD, is Associate Professor in the Graduate School of Social Service at Fordham University in New York. She has been active in the fields of domestic violence, aging and public welfare for more than 30 years. She is a John A. Hartford Foundation Geriatric Social Work Faculty Scholar and is the U.N. Representative to the International Network for the Prevention of Elder Abuse (INPEA). Dr. Brownell represents INPEA on the NGO Committee on Ageing of the United Nations and serves on the New York State Society on Aging Social Policy Committee. Her areas of research and practice are gerontology, elder abuse, and domestic violence, and she has a number of publications related to these topics.

About the Contributors

Marie Beaulieu, PhD, is Professor and Researcher at the University of Sherbrooke, Research Centre on Aging, Sherbrooke, Quebec, Canada.

L. René Bergeron, MSW, PhD, is affiliated with the Department of Social Work at the University of New Hampshire, Durham, New Hampshire.

Jacquelin Berman, PhD, is affiliated with the New York City Department for the Aging, New York, New York.

Patricia A. Bomba, MD, FACP, is Vice-President and Medical Director, Geriatrics, MedAmerica Insurance Company.

Maria L. Carpiac, MSW, is affiliated with the Department of Social Welfare at UCLA School of Public Policy and Social Research.

Carole A. Cohen, MD, is Associate Professor, Department of Psychiatry at the University of Toronto, Toronto, Ontario, Canada.

Christopher Dubble, MSW, is a Doctoral Student in Social Work at Fordham University, and Project Coordinator, Temple University Institute on Protective Services, Palmyra, Pennsylvania.

Deborah Heiser, PhD, is Researcher at the Isabella Geriatric Center, New York, New York.

Henry C. Hightower, PhD, is Partner in Hightower and Associates, and Emeritus Professor of Community and Regional Planning at the University of British Columbia.

Jill Hightower, MA, MJ, is Partner in Hightower and Associates, and Coordinator of the Older Women's Project for the BC/Yukon Society of Transition Houses.

Kerianne Lawson, MSW, MSG, is affiliated with the Beach Cities Health District.

Nancy Leclerc, MA, is a social worker and research professional with the Research Centre on Aging, Sherbrooke, Quebec, Canada.

Ailee Moon, PhD, is affiliated with the Department of Social Welfare at the UCLA School of Public Policy and Social Research.

Lisa Nerenberg, MSW, MPH, is Director of the Elder Abuse Prevention Program at the Goldman Institute on Aging, San Francisco, CA.

Elizabeth Podnieks, EdD, is affiliated with the Ryerson University School of Nursing, Toronto, Ontario, Canada.

Mebane E. Powell is affiliated with the New York City Department for the Aging, New York, New York.

Daniel A. Reingold is President and CEO of The Hebrew Home for the Aged, Riverdale, New York.

M. J. (Greta) Smith is a former Executive Director of the BC/Yukon Society of Transition Houses, and a coordinator of its Older Womens' Project. She established the Transition House in Quesnel BC.

Eleanor Spaziano, MSW, is affiliated with the VA Greater LA Healthcare System.

Foreword

Dr. Dobrof and I are pleased to present this special volume on elder abuse. Elder abuse, in all its manifestations, is not a new phenomenon. Considerable interest in it and concern for the victims of abuse existed in the U.S. prior to the passage of the Older Americans Act and the development of a network of publicly funded services for older persons. Today, there is a renewed interest in abuse of older persons, as an increasing number of health care and social service providers witness abuse among their patients and clients and join together to understand and respond.

Adults of any age, old or young, are victims of domestic violence but old age, itself, may bring a vulnerability, which exposes the older individual to risk of abuse. This is particularly true in areas of neglect, whether by others or self, and financial abuse. It is not uncommon for older persons to be pressured into handing over income to a younger relative, while a modus operandus for scam artists is, today, the targeting of older persons living alone who are viewed as easy 'hits.'

Elder abuse tends to cut across agency boundaries and frequently demands the involvement of different systems and professionals–lawyers, physicians, nurses, the courts, banks, and, of course, social workers. Haworth's published *Journals* include one devoted to elder abuse. It is read by those in all disciplines who are engaged on behalf of older abused persons. It is less likely to inform the social worker whose field of interest lies elsewhere and, yet, these social workers may be the first ones to come into contact with individual cases of elder abuse. It is for this reason that we have chosen to develop this special volume. It is intended to 'fill the gap' and to provide knowledge and skills to

[Haworth co-indexing entry note]: "Foreword." Mellor, M. Joanna. Co-published simultaneously in *Journal of Gerontological Social Work* (The Haworth Press, Inc.) Vol. 46, No. 3/4, 2006, pp. xxiii-xxiv; and: *Elder Abuse and Mistreatment: Policy, Practice, and Research* (ed: M. Joanna Mellor, and Patricia Brownell) The Haworth Press, Inc., 2006, pp. xix-xx. Single or multiple copies of this article are available for a fee from The Haworth Document Delivery Service [1-800-HAWORTH, 9:00 a.m. - 5:00 p.m. (EST). E-mail address: docdelivery@haworthpress.com].

xix

social workers in terms of assessing elder abuse when it is encountered and in knowing what, where and from whom, help may be sought. This collection is, however, more than a primer. The contributors are at the cutting edge within their specialties of policy, practice or research and present us with a wealth of information, equally useful to the novice and the expert.

M. Joanna Mellor, DSW
Co-Editor

Preface

Joanna Mellor and Patricia Brownell have done a superb job as co-editors of this special volume on Elder Abuse. As the reader will see, they have assembled articles on policy and practice issues and also there is attention to research, which, as is pointed out, continues to present particular challenges to social workers and other professionals.

Alas, psychological, social, and financial abuses continue to blight the lives of too many older people, and so this collection of articles is particularly timely. I wrote that last sentence, and was reminded of Congressional hearings years and years ago, at which one official (who shall remain nameless) reported to the House of Representatives Committee that the problem was less widespread than many advocates reported (claimed), and this official gave an estimate which was far lower than were the conventional estimates. And Congressman Mario Biaggi, who was chairing the hearings, thundered "Even one case of elder abuse is one too many!" Which, as the readers of this volume can imagine, brought the advocates who attended the hearing to their feet applauding to demonstrate their approval.

Rose Dobrof

[Haworth co-indexing entry note]: "Preface." Dobrof, Rose. Co-published simultaneously in *Journal of Gerontological Social Work* (The Haworth Press, Inc.) Vol. 46, No. 3/4, 2006, p. xxv; and: *Elder Abuse and Mistreatment: Policy, Practice, and Research* (ed: M. Joanna Mellor, and Patricia Brownell) The Haworth Press, Inc., 2006, p. xxi. Single or multiple copies of this article are available for a fee from The Haworth Document Delivery Service [1-800-HAWORTH, 9:00 a.m. - 5:00 p.m. (EST). E-mail address: docdelivery@haworthpress.com].

Introduction

Patricia Brownell, PhD

Elder abuse and neglect is a social problem of increasing concern to policymakers, practitioners, and researchers in the United States and around the world. Key policy concerns include the importance of improving the integration of service systems for elder abuse victims and their perpetrators. At the county level, adult protective service programs and law enforcement serve as front line interventions for the detection and intervention into adult abuse cases. However, conflicting mandates, definitions, and funding streams limit the effective coordination among these protective service systems.

POLICY ISSUES

Lisa Nerenberg provides a comprehensive overview of the history of community, state and national responses to the challenge of preventing and intervening in elder abuse and neglect situations. As Ms. Nerenberg notes, in spite of efforts on the part of researchers, policy makers at all levels of government, and program developers, the professional response to elder abuse remains fragmented and of uneven quality. Most recently, the federal Elder Justice Act provides the potential for a bi-partisan response to some of these policy questions. According to Christopher Dubble, the status of this important federal bill remains unknown in the Spring of 2005, as this volume moves into publication.

[Haworth co-indexing entry note]: "Introduction." Brownell, Patricia. Co-published simultaneously in *Journal of Gerontological Social Work* (The Haworth Press, Inc.) Vol. 46, No. 3/4, 2006, pp. 1-3; and: *Elder Abuse and Mistreatment: Policy, Practice, and Research* (ed: M. Joanna Mellor, and Patricia Brownell) The Haworth Press, Inc., 2006, pp. 1-3. Single or multiple copies of this article are available for a fee from The Haworth Document Delivery Service [1-800-HAWORTH, 9:00 a.m. - 5:00 p.m. (EST). E-mail address: docdelivery@haworthpress.com].

Available online at http://www.haworthpress.com/web/JGSW
doi:10.1300/J083v46n03_01

The issue of elder abuse and neglect has attracted international attention. It is gratifying that the UN is focusing attention on the social problem of elder abuse from a global perspective, emphasizing its human rights dimension. The Universal Principles for Older Persons address the importance of dignity for older adults: Principle #17 states: Older Persons should be able to live in dignity and security and be free of exploitation and physical or mental abuse. This principle is elaborated in the Madrid 2002 International Plan of Action on Ageing that came out of the Second World Assembly on Ageing. Issue 3 of the document provides a comprehensive definition of neglect, abuse and violence against older people, and includes the following objectives: (1) eliminate all forms of neglect, abuse, and violence of older persons (including elimination of risks to older women of all forms of neglect, abuse, and violence by increasing public awareness of and protecting older women from neglect, abuse and violence, especially in emergency situations) ; and (2) create support services to address elder abuse. Dr. Podnieks focuses on a key policy objective of the Madrid 2002 International Plan of Action on Ageing: addressing elder abuse and neglect by ensuring complete social inclusion of older adults in society.

PRACTICE ISSUES

A key concern of practitioners is strengthening the practice response to elder abuse and neglect. From a professional social work perspective, this can be challenging, as interdisciplinary collaboration is often essential to successfully prevent or address this tragic social issue. Dr. Bergeron explores the critical issue of self determination in working with elder abuse victims, particularly when victims may be nonvoluntary as is often the case with adult protective services clients. Dr. Bomba, a physician, proposes a practice tool that enables health care professionals to be more effective in detecting and assessing abuse and neglect among older adults. She emphasizes that often the signs and symptoms of elder abuse are overlooked by health care professionals, and as a result inadequate treatments or interventions are not provided. Daniel Reingold and Drs. Pat Brownell and Deborah Heiser discuss two intervention models for victims of elder abuse: a shelter program located in a nursing home, and a psycho-educational support group model. Dr. Carole Cohen addresses the widespread problem of financial abuse of older adults, including consumer fraud. Financial abuse is considered the most common form of elder abuse, and Dr. Cohen presents an overview of some successful initiatives developed to educate and protect older adults against this form of abuse.

RESEARCH

Researchers focused on elder abuse are challenged by definitional problems, ethical and methodological considerations, and the difficulties of gaining access to vulnerable subjects who may wish to conceal their mistreatment by loved ones and con artists. Dr. Marie Beaulieu presents the findings of a qualitative study intended to learn from practitioners more about issues and ethical dilemmas in work with elder abuse clients. Dr. Ailee Moon, with her colleagues Kerianne Lawson, Maria Carpiac, and Eleanor Spaziano, examine prevalence, types and intervention outcomes of elder abuse and neglect among ethnically and racially diverse veterans who are victims of elder abuse and neglect. Jill Hightower, M. J. (Greta) Smith, and Dr. Henry Hightower examine domestic violence of older women. Using a qualitative methodological approach, they explore the experiences of women age 50 years and older who have been abused by spouses and partners, comparing these experiences with those of younger battered women. Finally, Mebane Powell and Dr. Jacquelin Berman present findings of their study examining the relationship between dependency of abusers on their older adult victims, and the level of compliance with service plans by the older victims. Each of these studies applies different methodologies and research questions to diverse populations of elder abuse victims and their situations. In doing so, they expand our understanding of elder abuse and neglect in all its complexity, and strengthen the foundation on which effective policies and practice models and modalities can be developed.

Patricia Brownell, PhD
Co-Editor

Communities Respond to Elder Abuse

Lisa Nerenberg, MSW, MPH

SUMMARY. This article traces the development of services to prevent and treat elder abuse over a twenty-year time span. It begins by describing the various forms of elder abuse and the challenges they pose to service providers and program developers. Also described are abuse reporting statutes, the roles of various agencies involved in abuse investigations and responses, services commonly needed by victims, funding sources, and common impediments to service delivery. *[Article copies available for a fee from The Haworth Document Delivery Service: 1-800-HAWORTH. E-mail address: <docdelivery@haworthpress.com> Website: <http://www.HaworthPress. com> © 2006 by The Haworth Press, Inc. All rights reserved.]*

KEYWORDS. Elder abuse, prevention, services, service delivery, adult protective services, mandatory reporting, federal policy, state policy, mental capacity, multidisciplinary teams

[Haworth co-indexing entry note]: "Communities Respond to Elder Abuse." Nerenberg, Lisa. Co-published simultaneously in *Journal of Gerontological Social Work* (The Haworth Press, Inc.) Vol. 46, No. 3/4, 2006, pp. 5-33 ; and: *Elder Abuse and Mistreatment: Policy, Practice, and Research* (ed: M. Joanna Mellor, and Patricia Brownell) The Haworth Press, Inc., 2006, pp. 5-33. Single or multiple copies of this article are available for a fee from The Haworth Document Delivery Service [1-800-HAWORTH, 9:00 a.m. - 5:00 p.m. (EST). E-mail address: docdelivery@haworthpress.com].

Available online at http://www.haworthpress.com/web/JGSW
doi:10.1300/J083v46n03_02

In the twenty years since elder abuse first emerged into the public's consciousness, significant strides have been made in developing interventions, service programs and policy to prevent it. Researchers have attempted to measure the extent of the problem, establish profiles of victims and abusers, validate risk factors, assess victims' needs, and test the effectiveness of programs and services. States have enacted laws requiring professionals to report and designating public agencies to respond. Program developers at the local, state, and national levels have designed and tested a wide range of new services. Statutory and procedural innovations have made the civil and criminal justice systems more responsive.

Despite this progress, the professional response to elder abuse remains inadequate. Services are scarce, fragmented, of varying quality and poorly understood by the public, many professionals and the vulnerable elders they were created to serve. In many communities, coordination among law enforcement, social service agencies, courts, health care providers, and others is poor. Relatively few perpetrators are brought to justice, and many victims do not receive needed compensation, services or treatment.

This article provides an overview of what communities have done to address the needs of victims and vulnerable adults. It begins by briefly describing the various types of abuse and highlights the challenges each type poses to practitioners, program developers, and policy-makers. It describes services needed by victims, their families, and abusers; challenges to meeting these needs; and promising strategies and approaches.

WHAT IS ELDER ABUSE?

Definitions of elder abuse used by researchers, practitioners, and policy makers vary widely.[1] The definitions that follow are those of the author. They were drawn from multiple sources to illustrate the variety and complexity of abuse, highlight distinguishing features, and suggest some of the challenges each types poses to practitioners and program planners.

Physical abuse is intentionally or recklessly causing bodily injury, pain or impairment. Examples include striking, pushing, burning, and strangling elders, and using physical or chemical restraints. Assessing physical abuse against elders is often more difficult than assessments of younger victims because many common indicators of physical abuse and neglect, such as bruises, fractures, and weight loss, are often indistinguishable from accidental injuries or illness. The impact of violence against elders is often greater than for younger persons, and some jurisdictions have acknowledged this heightened lethality by enhancing penalties for violence against elders. Several specific forms of physical elder abuse have been the focus of special attention in recent years, including *elder domestic violence, homicide, suicide/homicides,* and *sexual assault.*

A first effort to explore *elder domestic violence* was initiated by AARP, which convened a 1992 symposium of researchers and practitioners in the fields of elder abuse and domestic violence to explore the scope and nature of violence against elderly women and how it was being addressed by both disciplines (AARP, 1993). The forum prompted a flurry of research and demonstration projects, which affirmed that domestic violence continues into old age and may be exacerbated by age-related conditions such as retirement, disability, and the changing roles of partners. Some women enter into violent relationships for the first time in advanced age. Regardless of their age at onset, elderly victims of domestic violence are not likely to receive needed services as a result of shortcomings in both networks. Domestic violence programs have not traditionally reached out to older women and lack the resources and expertise to meet their needs. Professionals who work with the elderly do not typically receive training to help them understand the dynamics of domestic violence, victims' help-seeking patterns, and effective approaches to ensuring safety and aiding recovery.

Homicides against elders pose special challenges to law enforcement agencies. They may be committed through suffocation, strangulation, starvation, neglect, over-medication, under-medication, drowning, causing someone to fall, poisoning, arson, or other means, and are likely to be mistaken for suicides, accidents, or deaths by natural causes. Many are staged to look that way. Some homicides are financially motivated; perpetrators may, for example, stand to inherit victims' estates or benefit in other ways from their victims' deaths. Serial killings involving predatory individuals who sought out employment in long term care facilities have also been reported. Some of these offenders claim to be "angels of mercy," who are helping patients die to relieve suffering, when, in fact, they are inflicting pain and suffering.

Elder homicide-suicides typically involve spouses or intimate partners who kill their partners and then commit suicide. Because these killings are likely to be prompted by the physical decline, hospitalization or institutionalization of either partner, they are often mistakenly assumed to be "double suicides" or "mercy killings" but closer scrutiny reveals that one partner was not a willing participant. Many suicide-homicides appear to be motivated by perpetrators' need to exercise power and control, and in one-third of cases, there is a history of domestic violence (Cohen, 1998).

Sexual abuse is non-consensual sexual contact of any kind with an older person. It includes rape; molestation; lewd or lascivious conduct; coercion through force, trickery or threats; or sexual contact with any person who lacks sufficient decision-making capacity to give consent. Elderly victims of sexual abuse are most often female and are likely to have impairments that make them dependent on others. Like many younger victims, they are likely to be embarrassed, afraid, humiliated and hesitant or unwilling to directly admit what has happened. Abusers include spouses and intimate partners, other relatives, paid caregivers and acquaintances. In long-term care facilities, abusers may be employees, contract workers, other residents and visitors.

Verbal or psychological abuse is the use of words, acts or other means to cause fear, humiliation, emotional stress, or anguish. Victims may be threatened with punishment, deprivation, or institutionalization. In long term care facilities, patients who complain may be threatened with eviction or other retaliatory acts. Other psychologically or verbally abusive acts include berating, infantalizing, humiliating, or ridiculing elders; cursing or making harsh commands; isolating them physically or emotionally; ignoring or failing to communicate with them; and promoting dependency. The impact of these forms of abuse is often difficult to assess because similar actions or words may be more traumatic to some individuals than others. Cultural norms and expectations also appear to significantly affect how these forms of abuse impact victims (Moon, 2000).

Financial abuse covers a broad spectrum ranging from simple theft to complex financial manipulations. It often involves the improper use of an older person's funds, property or resources, or inducing older people with diminished mental capacity to sign checks, deeds, wills or powers of attorney to benefit abusers. Seniors are also frequent targets of consumer fraud, telemarketing scams and "identity theft," which is the use of identifying information such as Social Security numbers to gain access to victims' finances or take out loans. "Sweetheart scams" are crimes in which offenders use deceptive romantic overtures to gain access to older people's assets. Residents in long-term care facilities may have personal property stolen by staff, visitors or other residents, or their family members may misuse or mismanage their assets or fail to pay their Medicaid share-of-cost, jeopardizing their care, damaging their reputations, or exposing them to adverse reactions by facility personnel.

Stopping financial abuse and recovering assets and property is extremely difficult. Proving that abuse occurred might require ascertaining what an elder with diminished mental capacity understood at an earlier point in time. Even when legal action is successful, few victims recoup misappropriated funds, which are likely to have been dissipated or hidden by offenders. The unlikelihood that victims will recover misappropriated property or be compensated for their losses prevents some victims from initiating or cooperating in legal proceedings even when the facts of a case suggest a high probability of success.

Neglect is the failure of any person who has responsibility for an elder to provide the level of care that a reasonable person in a like position would provide. It includes failure to provide medical, health, or mental health care; to assist in personal hygiene; to prevent malnutrition or dehydration; or to protect against health and safety hazards. Although neglect is sometimes viewed as less serious than acts of commission, its impact can be extremely serious, even leading to death. Failure to provide adequate nourishment to frail individuals can quickly lead to dehydration or malnutrition. When people who cannot turn by themselves are not assisted, they may develop pressure ulcers (also known as bedsores or decubitus ulcers), which are lesions caused by pressure that results in damage to the underlying tissue. When left untreated, pressure ulcers may cause sepsis. Failure to provide adequate assistance or medication can lead to accidents or illnesses becoming worse.

Persons at risk for neglect are individuals who rely on others as a result of frailty, or mental or physical disability. Perpetrators include family caregivers, paid attendants, long-term care facilities, and others who have a "duty" to provide care. The duty may be created by contractual arrangement (the caregiver is paid) or by virtue of a relationship (the parties are married). Determining responsibility is sometimes problematic because the extent to which family members are legally responsible for members has not been clearly established. In long term care facilities, neglect may be the result of individual employees' failure to perform their jobs or it may result from the facilities' failure to provide adequate staff coverage, training, or supervision.

Neglect may be unintentional or intentional. Unintentional neglect may occur when caregivers lack the necessary resources, physical strength, or stamina, emotional stability, maturity, or skills to meet elders' needs. Intentional neglect is willfully withholding needed care out of malice, indifference, or for financial gain (e.g., perpetrators want to hasten elders' death because they stand to inherit). Caregivers' motives or reasons for neglecting elders are critical considerations in shaping interventions.

Other forms are elder abuse include the *violation of basic human rights, abduction* and *abandonment*. Elders' human rights may be violated by spouses, other family members, individual caregivers or long term care facilities. Like all Americans, elders have the right to associate with whomever they choose, exercise choice and refuse psychotropic medications. They are further entitled to privacy and confidentiality. Residents of long-term care facilities are entitled to receive medical services and to choose their physicians. They are further protected against unnecessary physical restraint, involuntary seclusion, and separation from other residents.

Abduction includes taking elders from their residences and preventing them from returning using force, coercion, or undue influence. Perpetrators, who may include family members, caregivers, acquaintances, and others, may abduct elders to take possession of their homes or finances. They may remove elderly residents from long-term care facilities when it is not in the residents' best interest, it poses a danger, or when the elder lacks sufficient mental capacity to give consent and the person initiating the move lacks decision-making authority. Members of feuding families may abduct members because they don't believe other family members are providing adequate care. Intimate partners or spouses may abduct partners as a way of exercising power and control.

Abandonment is when people who are responsible for elders' care, including family members, paid caregivers or long term care facilities, willfully desert or forsake elders under circumstances in which reasonable people would continue to provide care. Elders may be left unattended in public settings or hospital emergency rooms. Caregivers may leave elders alone without adequate provisions, quit or move away without arranging for substitutes. Residents of long-term care facilities may be discharged with no place to go. Family members may leave older individuals in long-term care facilities and subsequently fail to visit or assist with care decisions.

All of the forms of abuse discussed above may be experienced by residents of long term care facilities as well as seniors living in the community. Abuse in facilities may be committed by family members, visitors, other residents and employees, or it may be the result of management practices, such as failure to provide adequate staff, or to screen or supervise employees. When abuse is committed by facilities' personnel, responsibility may rest with individual employees, supervisors, managers, administrators, or corporate entities.

COMMUNITY RESPONSES TO ABUSE AND NEGLECT

Communities began to respond to abuse in the early 1980s. The majority of states enacted laws mandating or encouraging professionals to report abuse, and professionals in many local communities organized coalitions or councils to assess local needs for training, community outreach, services, public policy, and service coordination.

Abuse Reporting Laws

Abuse reporting laws, which were closely patterned after child abuse reporting laws, enlist the help of professionals and the public to identify abuse and initiate investigations. The laws typically contain definitions of abuse and specify who must report, who *may* report, to whom reports are made, time requirements, what must be reported, penalties for failure to report, provisions for confidentiality and penalties for impeding investigations. Some state laws contain provisions for cross reporting among agencies authorized to conduct investigations, law enforcement, agencies that regulate long-term care facilities and others.

Adult Protective Services (APS)

Most states have designated adult protective service (APS) programs to receive, investigate and respond to abuse reports. APS dates back to the passage of Title XX of the Social Security Act in 1975, which permitted states to use funds, now known as Social Services Block Grants (SSBG), for specified purposes, which include advocacy and services for adults who, "as a result of physical or mental limitations, are unable to act in their own behalf, are seriously limited in the management of their affairs, are neglected or exploited, or who are living in unsafe or hazardous conditions."

The federal government provides little guidance to APS programs, and they vary widely across the country. Typically, when APS workers receive reports of abuse, they conduct home visits to assess the older or disabled person's risk, their capacity to give informed consent, and their need for medical, legal, financial or social services. Programs vary significantly with respect to the services they provide and their resources and sophistication. Some APS programs simply investigate reports, referring victims who need additional services to other community agencies, while others provide a comprehensive array of services including counseling, on-going financial management, emergency shelter and crisis intervention. They may also collect evidence and testimony to substantiate abuse, advocate on clients' behalf, and provide testimony in legal proceedings. Many APS programs lack adequate staff to meet community need, their workers do not receive specialized training, and the tools they use for assessing and responding to abuse are rudimentary. Other programs have extensive and on-going training for staff, 24-hour-a-day emergency response capability, state-of-the-art risk assessment tools, databases of clients and abusers, consultants to provide specialized expertise in such issues as medical forensics or financial abuse, formal appeals processes for alleged abusers, and protocols for interagency coordination.

APS services are voluntary, which means that elders and dependent adults can stop investigations and refuse interventions at any point. Under the following circumstances, however, workers typically initiate or make referrals for involuntary services:

- Elders and dependent adults who pose a danger to themselves or others, or who are "gravely disabled" (cannot meet their needs for food, clothing and shelter) as a result of mental illness, may be referred for psychiatric evaluations, treatment or hospitalization.
- Elders and dependent adults who lack sufficient mental capacity to understand and/or protect themselves against abuse, neglect, exploitation, or undue influence for reasons other than mental illness may be referred for probate guardianship. A few states have "protective custody," a procedure that allows extremely debilitated individuals who are at high risk to be removed from their homes for comprehensive assessments and follow up care.
- When the abuse constitutes criminal conduct, workers make referrals to appropriate law enforcement agencies.

OTHER AGENCIES THAT PLAY A ROLE IN INVESTIGATING ABUSE

Several other agencies play primary or supportive roles in responding to abuse reports. The involvement and responsibilities of the agencies listed below are determined by state and federal statutes and depend upon such factors as the type of abuse, its severity, whether the abuse constituted criminal conduct (and the type of crime), whether the abuse occurred in institutional settings or in the community, and whether institutions receive Medicare or Medicaid funding.

- *Local Law Enforcement*: Local police and sheriffs investigate crimes, apprehend suspects and present evidence. Police may also assist in securing and enforcing emergency protective orders and check on the well- being of frail isolated persons who are believed to be in danger.
- *Bureaus of Medicaid Fraud and Elder Abuse*: Typically located within offices of attorneys general, the bureaus investigate and prosecute fraud in the administration of Medicaid and the misappropriation of patient funds in facilities. They also review complaints of patient abuse and neglect when the facilities or their employees are responsible.
- *Long-Term Care Ombudsman Program (LTCOP)*: These federally mandated and funded programs protect the health, safety, welfare, and rights of elderly residents in long-term care facilities. The programs recruit and train volunteers to visit facilities and make themselves available to residents to discuss complaints of poor care. Ombudsmen report serious problems to state regulatory and licensing agencies and inform residents

and their families of available resources and remedies. They assist in relocating residents when facilities are forced to close down. In a few states, they are further mandated to investigate abuse and neglect reported in long-term care facilities under state reporting laws.

- *State Licensing Agencies*: Abuse and other problems occurring in long-term care facilities may also be reported to state agencies responsible for licensing and monitoring them.
- *Probate Court Investigators*: Some communities have probate court investigators who investigate proposed guardianships and monitor complaints of abuse by guardians.

SERVICES THAT MAY BE NEEDED BY VICTIMS OF ABUSE

Victims' service needs span a broad spectrum. Preventative services focus on lowering the risk of abuse, which may be accomplished by reducing vulnerable seniors' isolation and dependency, easing the strain on caregivers, strengthening caregiving systems, helping vulnerable persons plan and rehearse what they will do if abuse occurs, and enlisting the help of formal and informal supports to monitor potentially abusive situations. Stopping abuse and preventing its recurrence may require legal interventions to restrain abusers; removing victims from unsafe settings; providing information, support and encouragement to victims; and securing property. Services to help victims recover from abuse and neglect include medical treatment or health care, group or individual counseling, legal actions to recover property that has been misappropriated, credit counseling, and support services.

Specific services include those listed below. Most are provided by public or private nonprofit agencies, while others, including case management, counseling, legal services, mental health assessments, and support services, are also available from for-profit organizations. Their availability varies significantly across the country.

- *Shelters.* Elderly victims may need shelter in a variety of situations. Some require safe haven from abusers to avoid further victimization; for example, a victim may be particularly unsafe after filing for a restraining order. Others need shelter when they have been evicted from homes or apartments, abandoned by caregivers, when abusive caregivers have been fired or arrested, when essential utilities have been discontinued, or when their homes are unsafe or unhealthy as a result of abuse or neglect. A variety of shelter options have been designed, including rooms in battered women's shelters that have been adapted to meet the special needs of older women, temporary stays in residential care facilities or senior apartment houses, and free-standing shelters that have been designed specifically for victims of elder abuse.

- *Respite.* Respite care services provide relief to caregivers in several ways: Attendants, professionals or volunteers may come to elders' homes to give caregivers a break for a few hours, or the elders may be brought to special centers. Some skilled nursing facilities admit patients for longer periods.
- *Counseling.* Group or individual counseling may be needed to alleviate the immediate and long-term traumatic stress associated with abuse, provide emotional support, assist victims explore their options, and address such issues as co-dependence, depression, and diminished self-esteem.
- *Emergency funds* may be needed for food, emergency caregivers, mortgage payments, transportation, utilities, locks to secure victims' homes, court filing fees, repairs and relocation costs.
- *Legal assistance* may be needed to secure orders of protection, annul bogus marriages, sue for civil recoveries, create, or revoke powers of attorney, handle guardianships, etc.
- *Case management* is an approach to "brokering" or coordinating services for individuals who have multiple and changing care needs. Case managers perform comprehensive assessments of the older person's general health, mental capacity and ability to manage in the home and community. After completing the assessments, case managers develop "care plans," often in consultation with professionals from several disciplines, to meet clients' service needs and arrange for services. They also respond to problems or emergencies and conduct routine re-assessments to detect changes. Case management programs are increasingly gaining expertise in working with abuse victims, who often require services that fall outside the scope of traditional long-term care services.
- *Victim witness assistance programs,* which are usually located within prosecutors' offices, help victims whose cases are in the criminal justice system. They provide information to victims about the court process and the status of their cases; court accompaniment; and assistance securing compensation, restitution and community services.
- *Mental health assessments* are often needed to determine if elders are capable of meeting their basic needs, making decisions about services, entering into contracts, offering testimony, and protecting themselves against abuse. Assessments of alleged abusers' mental status are sometimes needed to determine if they pose a danger to others and need treatment. Assessments range from simple "mini-mental state exams" to comprehensive batteries of tests.

- *Support services* decrease vulnerability to abuse and neglect by enhancing the independence of elders with physical and cognitive limitations and reducing their reliance on others. Examples include daily money management, meals, attendant care, adult day centers, friendly visitors, and telephone reassurance programs.
- *Guardianship* is a legal proceeding in which courts appoint individuals or agencies to manage the personal and/or financial affairs of people who lack sufficient mental capacity to manage on their own and who are vulnerable to abuse, neglect, or other harm. There are two types of guardianships: "Guardianship of person" refers to the handling of an individual's personal needs such as medical care, food, clothing, and shelter; and "guardianship of estate (or property)" refers to the management of financial resources and assets. Guardianship is often the only alternative available for appointing surrogates for people who have lost decision-making capacity (and cannot, therefore, appoint surrogates themselves) or when less restrictive legal devices like trusts or powers of attorney have been misused. Guardians may be family members, professionals in private practice, private non-profit agencies, or public entities (called "public guardians").

MULTIDISCIPLINARY TEAMS

The diversity and complexity of abuse cases makes it unlikely that any single agency has all the resources, services or expertise needed to handle all types. For that reason, many communities have organized multidisciplinary teams (MDTs) to provide a forum for professionals from diverse disciplines and agencies to discuss difficult abuse cases; learn what services, approaches and resources are available from other agencies and disciplines; share information and expertise; identify and respond to systemic problems; and ensure offender accountability. Typically, teams include health and social service providers, law enforcement personnel, Ombudsmen, mental health care providers, physicians, advocates for persons with developmental disabilities, lawyers, domestic violence advocates, financial institutions, money managers, case managers, and many others.

In the last decade, specialized teams have emerged in response to the increasingly diverse and complex types of abuse being reported (Teaster & Nerenberg, 2004; Nerenberg, 2004). Several communities have formed Financial Abuse Specialist Teams (FASTs), which include members with expertise in such areas as real estate, insurance, banking practices, investments, trusts, estate and financial planning, and other financial matters. Because financial abuse may fall under the jurisdiction of state and federal law enforcement and regulatory agencies, FASTs are likely to include representatives from U.S. Attorneys' offices, the Federal Bureau of Investigation, the Federal Trade Commission, state bureaus of Medicaid fraud and abuse, and state regulatory agencies in addition to local law enforcement. A variation of the FAST model is the Rapid Response FAST, a model that was developed to respond quickly to financial emergencies, including situations in which clients' assets are in jeopardy. These teams tend to be small and include APS workers, public guardians, police, district attorneys, and city or county counsel. Team members may conduct joint interviews with clients within hours after a report is received so that immediate actions can be initiated to secure vulnerable assets and prevent further abuse.

Elder Fatality Review Teams, which were patterned after child and domestic violence fatality review teams, evaluate injuries and causes of death, attempt to distinguish accidental from non-accidental deaths, shed light on events leading up to deaths, identify systemic problems, and aid in prosecutions. Teams include coroners/medical examiners, law enforcement (local, state and, in some situations, federal), prosecutors, state agencies that oversee long-term care facilities, and others. Mental health professionals may provide guidance in evaluating the pre-death mental state of decedents to look for signs of suicide and interpret decedents' cognitive status prior to their deaths.

A few communities have developed teams with a medical focus. The teams, made up primarily of medical professionals, evaluate injuries and signs of neglect, assess cognitive functioning, interpret medical evidence or testimony, and provide testimony in court.

FUNDING FOR SERVICES TO PREVENT ABUSE

The primary sources of federal funding for elder abuse prevention services and education are the Social Services Block Grant (SSBG) and the Older American's Act (OAA). The SSBG supports the activities of APS units, and the OAA supports professional training, coordination of state and local social services systems, reporting hotlines, technical assistance for service providers, and public education.

Other sources of federal funding that are increasingly being used to serve elder abuse victims are the Victims of Crime Act (VOCA) and the Violence Against Women Act (VAWA). VOCA programs are administered by the Office for Victims of Crime. There are two programs that provide direct relief to victims, which are funded by federal criminals using fees, fines, and recoveries: Victims Compensation remunerates victims for crime-related expenses including shelter, counseling, funeral expenses, repairs, and loss of support. Victim Assistance provides funding to agencies for community-based services. Originally, VOCA programs only served victims of physical violence and required victims to cooperate with law enforcement. In recent years, VOCA revised its guidelines encouraging states to fund new services or expand existing services to victims of financial crimes and extending eligibility to clients whose cases were handled by APS as well as law enforcement. VOCA further encouraged states to promote the development of services to underserved groups, which include the elderly. As a result, states can now use VOCA funds to provide support for activities that address the immediate health and safety needs of victims of financial exploitation, including mental health/support counseling, respite care, and credit counseling, as well as for public information, outreach, advocacy and training for social service workers in recognizing and assisting victims of this abuse. Because states have discretion in the use of VOCA funds, some, but not all, have changed their priorities in response to the new regulations.

VAWA, through the Office on Violence Against Women, provides grants to assist states, tribal governments and local governments improve their law enforcement, prosecution and victim service responses to women who have been victims of violent crimes. It further provides training for judges, law enforcement personnel, prosecutors and the private bar to enhance their response to domestic violence, stalking and sexual assault victims. When the act was reauthorized in 2001, it identified elderly women as an underserved population and authorized funds for services and training focusing on elder abuse and sexual assault against the elderly and persons with disabilities. In 2002, funds were appropriated and awarded to law enforcement and prosecutorial agencies, professional associations, sexual assault and domestic violence coalitions, and others to improve the response to elderly victims. Additional grants were awarded in 2003.

The federal government has also promoted the development of state and local programs through research and demonstration projects, technical assistance, resource centers, and professional exchanges (U.S. Department of Justice Office of Justice Programs, 2000). The Administration on Aging (AoA), using OAA funds, has supported research to test the efficacy of abuse prevention services and funded demonstration projects to promote interagency coordination and develop services for older battered women. AoA also provided partial funding for a national incidence study on elder abuse (NCEA, 1998) and supports the National Center on Elder Abuse, which is operated by the National Association of State Units on Aging in collaboration with the National Adult Protective Services Association, the University of Delaware, the Commission on Law and Aging of the American Bar Association, and the National Committee for the Prevention of Elder Abuse. The Center operates the Clearing-house on Abuse and Neglect of the Elderly and a list serve, conducts profess-ional forums and events, produces technical assistance materials, and con-ducts small research studies.

The U.S. Department of Justice Office for Victims of Crime has also pro-vided funding for research and demonstration projects, technical assistance and training. These include grants to the National Sheriff's Association to pro-mote the development of TRIADs (coalitions of senior advocates, law en-forcement officials, and social service providers), the National Hispanic Council on Aging to develop culturally specific campaigns to combat finan-cial abuse, Oregon's Department of Human Services to develop materials on replicating its bank reporting project, and the Commission on Law on Aging of the American Bar Association to promote the development of elder death review teams. OVC has also convened several important national forums and focus groups to explore financial crimes, develop forensic expertise (U.S. De-partment of Justice, 2000), and promote interdisciplinary coordination (U.S. Department of Justice Office of Justice Programs, 2000). In addition to the grants it provides to local communities and states to develop training materi-als, the Office on Violence Against Women provides funds to the Wisconsin Coalition Against Domestic Violence to operate the National Clearinghouse on Abuse in Later Life.

Many states augment federal APS funding and provide additional funds for special projects such as outreach campaigns, training, and model projects. The extent to which states contribute abuse prevention efforts varies dramatically across the country.

CHALLENGES TO SERVING VICTIMS OF ELDER ABUSE

Although headway has been made, a variety of obstacles have impeded the development of elder abuse prevention programs and services. These range from inadequate resources to fundamental differences in how abuse is concep-tualized by various disciplines and interest groups, which have led to differ-ence in how they believe the problem needs to be addressed. This section illustrates some of the obstacles that communities and states have faced in de-veloping effective programs.

Lack of a Coordinated Federal Response

Because no federal agency has been designated to oversee or coordinate abuse reporting or to establish guidelines or standards for service delivery, states have struggled independently to design and implement reporting systems and service programs. This has led to wide variations across the country, and even within states, in how abuse is defined; eligibility for services; and how reported cases are assessed, prioritized, and responded to. Because no federal agency routinely collects information about abuse cases and current practices, there is no reliable data on which to develop a national profile of elder abuse or guide policy and service development. Specifically, program planners lack information on which to estimate the demand for services and the associated staffing needs and costs.

Inadequate Resources for APS and Other Services

Growing awareness about elder abuse, as well as the enactment of reporting laws, have led to dramatic increases in APS caseloads. The increasing complexity of cases and the expanded role APS programs are playing has further stretched resources. For example, APS programs are receiving more reports of sexual assault, concealed homicides, abuse in long-term care facilities, and complex forms of financial abuse, which call for labor-intensive investigations and follow up. In the past, the focus of APS investigations was to determine if vulnerable adults were in need of, and met eligibility criteria for, protective services. Greater emphasis on holding perpetrators accountable in recent years has meant that APS workers are now being called upon to provide evidence and testimony in civil and criminal proceedings, operate abuse registries and develop systems to ensure due process for abusers. As the "stakes" for committing abuse increase (e.g., perpetrators stand to be prosecuted or denied employment), workers need stronger investigative skills, and agencies must concern themselves with substantiation procedures, their liability for false claims, and how information about abusers can and should be used. Despite these added responsibilities, federal funding for SSBG remains relatively low and falls far short of that which goes to child protective services.

A possible explanation for the low funding levels and lack of leadership in APS is that the program has never achieved a high level of public recognition or support. Despite its pivotal role in abuse prevention, APS lacks visibility and is poorly understood by the public and many professionals. Advocacy organizations representing the populations APS serves, the elderly and disabled adults, have not advocated on APS' behalf. In contrast, child protective services are highly visible, well-defined and regulated, placing APS at a disadvantage when it comes to advocating for a fair share of SSBG dollars.

Some states have changed their formulas for distributing discretionary federal funding, including SSBG, to achieve greater parity for abused elders. As described earlier, some have devoted more VOCA funds to programs that serve elderly victims. Despite these efforts, funding for services to victims of elder abuse falls far short of that devoted to other forms of abuse. It has been estimated that the federal government spends $153.5 million on programs addressing issues of elder abuse, compared to the $520 million it spends on domestic violence and $6.7 billion on child abuse prevention (U.S. Senate Special Committee on Aging, 2002).

Administrative Barriers

The fact that services to abused elders are partially funded by multiple federal programs makes it difficult for agencies to create comprehensive and seamless service systems, raising the risk that victims will fall between the cracks of the service delivery system. For example, VAWA funds are intended for programs that serve elderly victims of domestic violence and sexual assault, excluding male victims and victims of other forms of abuse. VOCA funds have historically only served victims of violent crimes. As described earlier, changes in federal regulations permit states to use VOCA funds to serve victims of other forms of abuse, but not all states have done so. Older Americans Act funds are primarily for outreach and education. Agencies wishing to provide a comprehensive range of education and services to all victims of elder abuse must, therefore, draw from multiple funding streams, each with its own administrative requirements and policies, eligibility criteria, funding cycles, and bureaucracy.

Ideological or "Cultural" Differences Among Agencies or Disciplines

Divergent perspectives and ideologies may cause strains and tensions that impede cooperation or coordination among the various disciplines that have a role to play in abuse prevention. For example, domestic violence theory and practice is grounded in feminist ideology, attributing domestic violence to society's attitudes about and treatment of women. Some elder abuse programs have attempted to make domestic violence services and resources available to victims whose situations do not meet the traditional definition of domestic violence,[2] raising objections from domestic violence programs. Conflicts have also arisen between the elder abuse and younger disabled communities with respect to such issues as whether Medicaid beneficiaries should be permitted to use public funds to hire family members or friends as personal care attendants and how problems, including abuse by caregivers, should be handled. Advocates for persons with disabilities have historically advocated for greater control over hiring and firing decisions, while many advocates for the elderly believe that seniors' vulnerability to coercion, threats and undue influence places them at an unfair advantage when it comes to exercising their roles as health care consumers. Heightened focus on prosecution in recent years has raised concern among some health and social service providers that the "criminalization" of elder abuse will discourage families from seeking needed help.

Mental Capacity, Consent, and Undue Influence

Clients' mental capacity and their ability to make decisions are pivotal considerations in serving victims of elder abuse. They dictate whether involuntary measures are needed and determine the type of interventions that are available and appropriate. From professionals' first contact with vulnerable clients, they are faced with critical decisions regarding clients' capacity to refuse or accept help. While this is true for anyone who works with persons with disabilities, the "stakes" are typically higher when abuse is alleged and misjudgments about clients' ability to give consent may result in abuse, neglect, or exploitation.

Assessing mental capacity is complex for many reasons. Capacity may fluctuate widely and is affected by such variables as time of day, nutritional status and stress. In addition, mental capacity is made up of many mental skills and abilities such as memory, abstract thinking, and reasoning. The type and extent of capacity that is needed for making decisions depends on the type of decision in question. For example, a person who is capable of deciding whom they want to leave their assets to may be incapable of weighing the benefits of a reverse annuity mortgage. Professionals have little guidance when assessing capacity for many of the decisions commonly required in abuse cases. These include such pivotal decisions whether an elder has sufficient capacity to consent to (or refuse) an abuse investigation.

Further complicating matters is the fact that one's ability to make decisions may also be impaired by psychological manipulation or control exerted by others. Undue influence refers to the psychological control that stronger people exert over weaker people to get them to do things that they would not have done otherwise. Manipulators may endear themselves to vulnerable persons to get them to comply with their demands. Victims who are under the influence of abusers may refuse help because they are unaware that they are being manipulated.

Impediments to Prosecution

Much has been written in recent years about the difficulties involved in prosecuting crimes against the elderly. Barriers that have been identified include victims' unwillingness or inability to participate in criminal proceedings as a result of disability, shame, fear, or not wanting to see perpetrators (particularly family members) punished. Many professionals are reluctant to report abuse to law enforcement because they want to respect clients' wishes or do not fully understand the criminal justice system. In financial abuse cases, key evidence is likely to be in the hands of perpetrators or financial institutions.

When cases are reported to law enforcement, the outcomes are often disappointing. Elder abuse is not seen as a priority within most law enforcement agencies; this is particularly true of certain forms of abuse including financial exploitation, neglect and abuse in long-term care facilities. Few law enforcement officials and prosecutors have training or experience working with victims who have cognitive or communication impairments, or who have co-dependent or enmeshed relationships with their offenders, making them reluctant witnesses. Persistent beliefs that certain types of abuse, including the misuse of powers of attorney, are strictly civil matters, prevents some financial abuse cases from being filed or investigated.

Another impediment to prosecution is lack of forensics markers and expertise (Dyer, Connolly, & McFeeley, 2003). As described earlier, differentiating the signs and symptoms of abuse and neglect from accidental injuries, disease or other factors can be extremely complicated. More research is needed on such topics as bruising, falls, pressure ulcers, weight loss, nutritional deficits, and other factors to identify patterns of abuse.

Victims also lack incentives to participate in the criminal justice process. Coming to court can be a traumatic experience, particularly to frail older people who are likely to be treated insensitively. It can also be emotionally distressing to recount traumatic incidents or confront offenders. In addition, elderly victims are unlikely to receive restitution for financial losses, assistance by victim advocates, compensation for crime related expenses, or services to help them recover from crimes.

Service Gaps

Despite the progress that has been made in designing services and interventions, few, if any, communities have all the services that are likely to be needed by abused elders. Even when services exist, they may be in short supply. Several notable areas of need include surrogate decision-makers for abused or vulnerable elders, culturally specific programs and services for offenders.

Surrogate decision makers may be needed when abused or vulnerable elders lack sufficient decision-making capacity to act on their own behalf. In many cases, the only way to obtain surrogate decision-making authority over someone who has already lost capacity (and who has not executed an advance directive such as a durable power of attorney prior to the onset of incapacity) is guardianship, which is costly, stigmatizing, and restrictive. Although advocates have called for less restrictive alternatives, few communities have any. Examples of situations in which less restrictive alternatives may be appropriate are when decision-making authority is needed for single actions, such as revoking a power of attorney, for limited periods of time, or in emergencies. Promising areas for exploration include limited guardianships, time-limited protective placements, or ethics committees.

Although few studies have looked at cultural variations in elder abuse or how these differences affect the service needs of victims and their families, the existing research and practice experience suggests a need for culturally specific approaches (Tatara, 1999). Programs are needed that reflect cultural variations with respect to how abuse is perceived, the roles and expectations of family members, attitudes toward law enforcement and the service delivery system, confidentiality, immigration status, eligibility for services, and the heightened caregiving responsibilities that are common to several groups.

Few programs or services exist for abusers and would-be abusers. Notable exceptions include a self-assessment guide to help caregivers identify their own risk of becoming abusive, which was created by the Office of Geriatric Medicine/Gerontology at Northeastern Ohio Universities. Lifespan of Rochester, New York started the nation's first group for offenders. The program raises members' awareness about the impact of their actions on victims and changes culturally-derived attitudes.

MEETING THE CHALLENGE: INNOVATIONS AND BEST PRACTICES

Innovators across the country have demonstrated ingenuity and creativity in addressing many of the obstacles that have impeded service development. This section describes a few areas in which progress has been most evident. These include community responses to financial abuse and domestic violence, improving access to courts, the prosecution of abuse cases, preventative interventions and developing forensics expertise.

Preventing Financial Abuse

Effectively preventing financial abuse requires a multifaceted approach that reduces vulnerability, stops abuse and prevents its recurrence, secures vulnerable assets, and recovers property that has been lost.

Vulnerability to financial abuse may stem from diminished mental capacity, inexperience handling finances or susceptibility to undue influence. When trustworthy helpers assist vulnerable individuals pay bills, write checks, and make bank deposits, it can significantly reduce the risk of abuse. Although the potential of daily money management (DMM) to reduce the risk of abuse has long been acknowledged, social service agencies have been reluctant to provide the service as a result of difficulties obtaining insurance for workers and volunteers, concerns about liability and logistical challenges.

Several prominent organizations have attempted to overcome these problems. The Reingold Institute at the Brookdale Center on Aging of Hunter College developed a training and technical assistance program to encourage agencies to offer the service. AARP recruits and trains members to provide DMM for low income and disabled persons under the supervision of state and local agencies, which have cooperative agreements with AARP. AARP also provides technical assistance to its partner agencies, as well as insurance for volunteers. Massachusetts was the first state to implement the AARP program statewide in collaboration with the state's 27 "Aging Services Access Points" (ASAPs), which provide case management to low income seniors. Bank employees have been recruited as volunteers in some communities, with some banks allowing employees to provide volunteer service during normal working hours under their Community Reinvestment Act requirements (a Congressional act that encourages depository institutions to help meet the credit and financial service needs of the communities they serve).

Because DMM is a labor intensive service (money managers may need to disburse cash to clients on a weekly or biweekly basis) methods to increase efficiency have also been explored. Southern California Presbyterian Homes, a provider of supportive and low income housing, developed a DMM program for its residents after discovering that many of them were having trouble managing their financial affairs. The program operates in conjunction with a multiservice senior center and the University of Southern California. UC is evaluating the program to measure its impact, shed light on client characteristics associated with need for the service, and provide insight into the special needs of immigrant and non-native English speaking clients (a relatively high proportion of the program's clients are Armenian or Hispanic).

Abuse of powers of attorney has been the focus of attention as reports of agents using their powers to exploit rather than protect become increasingly common. Historically, there has been little oversight to ensure that persons signing powers have the requisite legal capacity and that agents are using the powers for their intended purposes. Initiatives to prevent this type of abuse have included education to consumers, training to lawyers and other professionals in crafting powers that offer maximum protection, and statutory reform. In 1993, the Government Law Center at the Albany Law School developed recommendations for how states can improve protection; more recently, the National Conference of Commissioners on Uniform State Laws, an organization of lawyers, judges and law professors, revised its Uniform Durable Power of Attorney Act to strengthen safeguards. For example, it recommends that powers expressly state (rather than imply) gift-making authority and that divorce or annulment should revoke a spouse-agent's authority.

Several communities have acknowledged a need for specialized expertise to help abuse investigators distinguish fraudulent from legitimate financial transactions, prevent losses, build cases for court, and recover losses. Innovative approaches include Oregon's Retiree Response Technical Team, which recruits retired bank personnel as volunteers to help protective service workers investigate financial abuse reports. APS in San Francisco established a specialized financial abuse unit; workers receive special training in financial abuse and work closely with the fraud unit of the Police Department. Under a pilot project conducted by Temple University's Institute on Protective Services, forensic accountants are made available to adult protective service agencies, police and district attorneys to assist with financial abuse investigations, write reports and serve as expert witnesses.

Communities are increasingly enlisting the help of financial institutions in identifying and reporting abuse and educating the public about the problem. This approach was first piloted by the Massachusetts Executive Office of Elder Affairs in collaboration with the Executive Office of Consumer Affairs, the Attorney General's Elderly Protection Project, and the Massachusetts Bank Association. Together, the groups developed procedures and guidelines for reporting and investigating abuse. Banks are provided with training for their personnel and informational materials for their customers. A similar program, the Oregon Bank Reporting Project, received funding from the U.S. Department of Justice Office for Victims of Crime to develop a kit for replicating its program, which has been disseminated nationally.

Improving the Response to Elderly Victims of Domestic Violence

In the last decade, many communities have adapted techniques, approaches and services commonly used in the field of domestic violence for older women. They have created age-appropriate shelters, support groups for older women, counseling programs and cross training for personnel of both domestic violence and elder abuse prevention programs.

The state of Wisconsin has, for many years, been a leader in promoting collaboration between the elder abuse and domestic violence networks. Its Bureau of Aging and Long Term Care Resources offered small grants to develop or improve services for older abused women and required counties to include representatives from domestic violence programs on interdisciplinary teams to be eligible for special direct service dollars.

Improving Court Access

Several communities have addressed the multiple obstacles that prevent many elderly victims from coming to court. The Elder Justice Center of the Thirteenth Judicial Circuit Court in Tampa, Florida was designed to assist elderly victims of financial abuse, domestic violence and consumer fraud negotiate the court system. A case manager explains the court system to victims, describes what will happen to perpetrators, arranges for needed services such as transportation or court accompaniment, and, when necessary, assists in making special arrangements such as videotaping testimony. Case managers may also request victim compensation or assist victims file for orders of protection using forms that have been reproduced in large typeface. The case manager also maintains an extensive directory of community services and makes referrals, following up to ensure that clients' needs are met. A second center has opened in West Palm Beach. A similar project, which is currently being carried out in Alameda County, has established a separate calendar for elders seeking restraining orders and schedules all cases in the late morning to accommodate elders. In some situations, when elders are unable to appear in court, the proceedings are conducted in chambers, with a judge issuing orders by telephone.

Improving Prosecution Rates

Among the most dramatic changes in the field of elder abuse prevention in recent years is the increasing number of abuse cases that are prosecuted. A variety of procedural and statutory innovations have helped to accomplish this. Procedural innovations include specialized elder abuse units within police departments and prosecutors' offices, legal centers that facilitate coordination between the civil and criminal justice systems, coordinating councils and multidisciplinary teams that promote exchange between law enforcement and other networks, and the use of vertical prosecution (a single attorney handles a case from the beginning to the end of a prosecution). Statutory innovations that have been implemented in some states include penalty enhancements for offenders who target the elderly, exceptions to hearsay restrictions, and provisions that make it easier to prosecute family members and others who are in positions of trust.

A variety of training initiatives, many of which are supported by federal funds, have enhanced law enforcement officers' and prosecutors' expertise in working with elderly victims and people with disabilities, including those who are reluctant or ambivalent about participating in the criminal justice process.

They are further gaining skills in building cases involving the misuse of civil instruments.

A few innovative programs have attempted to improve restitution recovery rates, thereby increasing incentives for victims to report abuse to police. Colorado conducted a pilot project that employed collections investigators in the court system to see that victims received court-ordered restitution. A review of the state's restitution statutes led to revisions, which include the requirement that criminal restitution be considered after conviction for any felony, misdemeanor, petty offense or traffic misdemeanor offense (USDOJ, 2002).

Building Forensics Expertise

Initiatives to meet the need for improved forensics expertise have emerged at the federal, state and local levels. At the national level, the U.S. Department of Justice convened a 2000 roundtable of researchers, practitioners and policy makers who described the current state of the art and challenges involved in identifying and substantiating abuse and neglect. The group called for research to establish abuse "markers," evidence-based data to support findings of abuse, clearinghouses of forensics experts who are available to testify or consult in cases, and databases of documented findings that can be used in the prosecution of abuse and neglect. A subsequent meeting was held in 2004 to review progress.

States and local communities are contributing to the forensics knowledge base by forming elder death review teams, providing training and consultation in forensics to APS workers and other professionals, conducting research and providing opportunities for professional exchange between medical and legal professionals.

The first elder death review teams were organized in the early 2000s. In 2002, the Commission on Law and Aging at the American Bar Association received funding from the U.S. Department of Justice Office for Victims of Crime to promote the development of local and state-level elder death review teams. Five sites were selected to receive technical assistance in developing teams.

At the state level, Arkansas passed the first state law in 1999 requiring nursing homes to report all deaths to the local coroner. In Pulaski County, over 2000 nursing home deaths were investigated, resulting in 100 cases being referred to the state's Attorney General for suspicion of abuse. In 2001, the California legislature called for the development of a medical forensic form to include instructions, guidance and examination protocols for examining victims of elder and dependent adult abuse and neglect. The form, which was developed by the Medical Training Center at the University of California at Davis, is currently being piloted.

At the local level, the Vulnerable Adult Specialist Team (VAST) of the University of California at Irvine College of Medicine is currently conducting research on bruising and provides consultation to community professionals in abuse cases. VAST also performs medical and cognitive evaluations, conducts home assessments, provides expert testimony in court cases, and provides training to medical residents. A similar program, the Texas Elder Abuse and Mistreatment (TEAM), is operated by the Baylor College of Medicine, the Harris County Hospital District, and Texas' APS program.

Reducing the Risk of Abuse and Neglect

Clearly, risk reduction and early intervention are the preferred approaches to abuse prevention. Several communities, states, and agencies have focused on developing risk reduction strategies. These include providing better screening of workers and strengthening family caregiving support systems.

Several states have enacted laws calling for long-term care facilities and licensed home care programs to conduct criminal background checks of potential employees (Nerenberg, 2002). Criminal records, which typically include police arrest reports, prosecution data, court determinations and records from corrections departments, are kept by both state and federal law enforcement agencies. The Federal Bureau of Investigation (FBI) collects information from all states and can provide information to local and state agencies about crimes committed outside their states. A few states allow potential employers of in-home care providers to obtain criminal background information on independent contractors and a few require that checks be performed.

An innovative, culturally specific program aimed at helping families develop plans for caregiving and resolve problems was developed by the Family Support Center of Jamestown S'klallam with funding from Administration on Aging's Native American Caregiver Support Program. The program uses "family group conferencing," a restorative justice approach that assumes that if families are involved and provided with adequate information, they can develop appropriate plans to deal with their own problems. This is accomplished through "talking circles" of 12 to 15 people who are chosen by the elder and typically include friends, family members and spiritual leaders. Although an administrator meets with service providers to discuss their concerns about the elders' health and safety prior to the circle, no more than one service provider is present during conferences at a time. Families referred to the Center may be experiencing stress as a result of burnout, problems coordinating services, and addressing end-of-life issues. The circles, which typically take five or six hours, are based on the "medicine wheel" concept. Members consider the four aspects of life in developing plans of care: the emotional, physical, spiritual, and social. The model is being tested with both Indian and non-Indian families. Tribes across the state have received training and a replication manual will be developed.

Strengthening APS

In recent years, new and existing organizations at the federal, state and local levels have begun to advocate more forcefully for APS. The National Adult Protective Services Association, a partner in the National Center on Elder Abuse, collects national data on APS clients and administration and supports federal legislation, including the Elder Justice Act (see below).

At the state level, several states, including Ohio and Wisconsin, have engaged in ambitious initiatives to evaluate and extend their protective service programs. The Wisconsin Department of Health and Family Services launched the Adult Protective Services Modernization Project in 1990 to examine the state's reporting system, services, laws and regulations and to recommend ways to improve the state's response. As the result of an aggressive statewide advocacy campaign spearheaded by county APS administrators in California, the state passed legislation in 1998, giving California its first comprehensive APS system along with sizeable increases in state general funds to cover the costs of the enhanced program.

State and local APS programs have also developed 24-hour emergency response systems, refined their approaches to risk assessment and case monitoring, developed databases of offenders, designed and tested a variety of new services, launched outreach campaigns, and enacted progressive management practices.

Advocacy

Comprehensive and coherent public policy is the goal of several national and state initiatives. In December of 2001, the National Center on Elder Abuse convened the first national summit on elder abuse with support from the Administration on Aging and Department of Justice. Experts from around the country adopted 21 recommendations, which included as priorities: a nationwide structure for abuse prevention activities; a national strategic communications program; improving the legal system's response to abuse; a comprehensive education and training curriculum; mental health services for the elderly; a General Accounting Office study of service needs; a national APS resource center to promote professional competence and service development; a research institute to oversee research, data collection, and program evaluation; and an Executive Order directing federal agencies, and inviting Governors, to review policies related to elder abuse.

In February of 2002, Senator John Breaux, ranking member of the Senate Special Committee on Aging, and Sen. Orrin Hatch, chairman of the Senate Judiciary Committee introduced the Elder Justice Act (HR 333). In June of the following year, the House introduced a companion measure, H.R. 2490, which is identical to the Senate version. The act establishes a national structure for administering abuse prevention programs and mechanisms for coordinating the activities of the multiple federal agencies involved in prevention. It further establishes a federal base for Adult Protective Services (APS) and ensures greater uniformity and consistency in funding. Dual "Offices of Elder Justice" within the Departments of Health and Human Services and Justice are proposed to oversee programs, grant-making, policy and technical assistance. The act further calls for research and data collection, establishing as priorities studies to ascertain the incidence and prevalence of abuse; reveal the effectiveness of interventions; identify community strategies to make elders safer; and reveal the costs of multi-disciplinary efforts. It calls for the creation of forensic centers, resource centers, a library and a data repository to collect information about abuse and promising practices for preventing it, professional training, the development of model statutes, and technical assistance.

Shortly after the introduction of the Elder Justice Act, a coalition of national, regional, state and local advocacy groups and concerned citizens, the Elder Justice Coalition, was formed to promote public understanding and support for the act. The National Committee for the Prevention of Elder Abuse is the lead agency for the organization.

Several states and counties have replicated NCEA's summit. In October of 2003, Washington County, Oregon, held a regional summit, which drew 100 legislators, prosecutors, district attorneys, law enforcement officials, APS workers and advocates. The group discussed eight areas of need, including better security checks for people who work with seniors, standards for guardians and conservators, and the "fast tracking" of civil and criminal elder abuse cases. New York convened a statewide event in 2004, producing its own action agenda.

CONCLUSION

The field of elder abuse emerged on the heels of major national initiatives to create a community-based long term care network. The goal of this network is to promote the independence of frail elders living in the community and avoid unnecessary institutionalization. To a great extent, elder abuse exposes the shortcomings of this network, revealing what can happen when community based caregiving systems are inadequate and fail to protect vulnerable elders against predatory individuals or businesses, negligent caregivers, greedy or troubled family members, or systemic failures. As communities mobilize to address elder abuse, they are further discovering critical failures by institutions that were created to protect all citizens, including law enforcement, the courts, domestic violence programs, consumer protection agencies, the health and mental health systems, financial institutions and others. More recently, they have revealed serious shortcomings in institutional care as well.

Creating effective community responses to elder abuse is not limited to launching new programs and services. Rather, it requires the sustained and systematic evaluation and monitoring of myriad programs and systems of care to ensure that elders have access. It involves shoring up existing programs to accommodate elders' special needs, promoting coordination and collaboration among diverse disciplines and networks, building consensus about how to best serve abused elders, and promoting public policy that supports and facilitates service delivery. Achieving these goals will require further research, the ongoing testing of promising practices, technical assistance to help communities implement programs as their effectiveness is demonstrated, public education, professional training and advocacy at the local, state, and national levels. More importantly, it will require a strong commitment by policymakers and the public.

The burgeoning elderly population has been touted as an incentive or rationale for heightened attention to elder abuse prevention. In recent years, the rights of persons with disabilities to remain in the community whenever possible has been adjudged to be a civil right (Olmstead Decision[3]), further heralding the need for greater protections for society's most vulnerable members. Clearly, today's successes and failures will have resounding impact in the next few decades.

NOTES

1. State-specific definitions are typically contained in elder and dependent adult reporting laws and criminal statutes. Definitions relating to abuse in long-term care facilities are likely to be found in business or professional, health and safety, or government codes.

2. Domestic violence is assaultive and coercive conduct used by men to exercise power and control over their female intimate partners using a variety of tactics.

3. A Supreme Court case brought by two Georgia women who were living in state-run institutions even though professionals had determined that they could be ap-

propriately served in community settings. The plaintiffs charged that continued institutionalization was a violation of their rights under the Americans with Disabilities Act (ADA). The court ruled in their favor, affirming that unjustified isolation constitutes discrimination based on disability. In response, the Department of Health and Human Services directed states to increase their efforts to enable people with disabilities to live in the community and provide them with more opportunities to exercise informed choice.

REFERENCES

AARP. (1993). *Abused elders or older battered women? Report on the AARP forum.* Washington, DC: AARP Women's Initiative.

Cohen, D. (1998). Homicide-suicide in older persons. *American Journal of Psychiatry, 155,* 390-396.

Dyer, C.B., Connolly, M.T., & McFeeley, P. (2003). The clinical and medical forensics of elder abuse and neglect. In R.J. Bonnie & R.B. Wallace (Eds.), *Elder Mistreatment: Abuse, Neglect, and Exploitation in an Aging America.* (pp. 339-381). Washington, DC: The National Academies Press.

Heisler, C.J., & Steigel, L. (2002). Enhancing the justice system's response to elder abuse: Discussions and recommendations of the "Improving Prosecutions" working group of the national policy summit on elder abuse. *Journal of Elder Abuse & Neglect, 14*(4), 31-54.

Moon, A. (2002). Perceptions of elder abuse among various cultural groups: Similarities and differences. *Generations, 24*(2), 75-80.

National Center on Elder Abuse. (1998). *The national elder abuse incidence study.* Report prepared for the Administration on Aging an Administration for Children and Families in collaboration with Westat, Inc., Washington DC: Author.

Nerenberg, L. (2002). The national policy summit issue briefs. *Journal of Elder Abuse & Neglect, 14*(4), 71-104.

Nerenberg, L. (2002). *Preventing elder abuse by in-home helpers.* San Francisco: Institute on Aging.

Nerenberg, L. (2004). *Multidisciplinary elder abuse prevention teams: A new generation.* Retrieved July 21, 2004 from the National Center on Elder Abuse Web site: http://www.elderabusecenter.org/pdf/publication/EldAbs_complete.pdf

Pillemer, K.A., & Suitor, J.J. (1992). Violence and violent feelings: What causes them among family caregivers? *Journal of Gerontology: Social Sciences, 47*(4), 165-172.

Tatara, T. (1999). *Understanding elder abuse in minority populations.* Philadelphia: Taylor & Francis.

Teaster, P.B., & Nerenberg, L. (2003). *A national look at elder abuse multidisciplinary teams:* Retrieved July 21, 2004 from the National Center on Elder Abuse Web site: http://www.elderabusecenter.org/pdf/publication/mdt.pdf

U.S. Department of Justice. (2000). *Elder justice: Medical forensic issues related to elder abuse and neglect roundtable discussion.* Washington, DC: Author.

U.S. Department of Justice, Office of Justice Programs (1998). *The focus group on crime victimization of older persons: Recommendations to the Office of Justice Programs.* Washington, DC: Author.

U.S. Department of Justice, Office of Justice Programs (2000). *Our aging population: Promoting empowerment, preventing victimization, and implementing coordinated interventions. Symposium report of the proceedings.* Washington, DC: Author.

U.S. Senate Special Committee on Aging. (2002). *Protecting America's seniors: A history of elder abuse, neglect, and exploitation. Executive summary.* Retrieved July 21, 2004 from Senator John Breaux's Web site: http://breaux.senate.gov/aging/elder justice/wpsummary.html#N_9_

A Policy Perspective
on Elder Justice Through APS
and Law Enforcement Collaboration

Christopher Dubble, MSW

SUMMARY. The policy issues involved in the social problem of elder victimization could fill volumes. Even the policy issues involved in the new concept of elder justice are multi-faceted. Through the lens of a policy analysis perspective, the history, ideologies, politics, social movements, and economics of policies that promote the collaboration between adult protective services and law enforcement are examined. The analysis of state and local policies as well as a promising federal legislative initiative will, hopefully, help policy advocates understand from where the movement toward collaboration between adult protective services and law enforcement has come as well as where it may be headed. *[Article copies available for a fee from The Haworth Document Delivery Service: 1-800-HAWORTH. E-mail address: <docdelivery@haworthpress.com> Website: <http://www.HaworthPress.com> © 2006 by The Haworth Press, Inc. All rights reserved.]*

KEYWORDS. Abuse, elder justice, adult protective services, neglect, exploitation, multi-disciplinary

---

[Haworth co-indexing entry note]: "A Policy Perspective on Elder Justice Through APS and Law Enforcement Collaboration." Dubble, Christopher. Co-published simultaneously in *Journal of Gerontological Social Work* (The Haworth Press, Inc.) Vol. 46, No. 3/4, 2006, pp. 35-55 ; and: *Elder Abuse and Mistreatment: Policy, Practice, and Research* (ed: M. Joanna Mellor, and Patricia Brownell) The Haworth Press, Inc., 2006, pp. 35-55. Single or multiple copies of this article are available for a fee from The Haworth Document Delivery Service [1-800-HAWORTH, 9:00 a.m. - 5:00 p.m. (EST). E-mail address: docdelivery@haworthpress.com].

Mention the words elder justice in conversation with lay people and experts alike and expect to receive, in return, quizzical glares communicating skepticism as to whether the term is part of the American vernacular. To date, the ideas that the term represents have been advanced only by a small cohort of advocates and professionals in the field of elder victimization or more commonly referred to as elder abuse and neglect. While certainly the notion of elder justice is defined differently by different people, there is a clear sense among a bantam and growing contingent, comprised of politicians, researchers, practitioners and advocates, that elder justice, at least in part, must include policies to mandate collaborative relationships between the adult protective service (APS) and law enforcement systems when victimization rises or has the potential to rise to a criminal standard. These advocates believe that the implementation of such policies is an effectual and essential method of intervention to meet the multi-faceted needs of older victims and contribute to the greater good of the communities where the victims reside.

Today, federal legislation with the potential to advance the relationships between law enforcement and APS in combating elder victimization has many who favor this conceptualization of elder justice quite excited. The legislation is titled the Elder Justice Act. The Act is the first federal effort to propose policies and funding that bring the two systems together to provide both service and justice for older victims. Presently, older victims in most jurisdictions are only provided with half of the equation, at best. As put in the press release announcing the introduction of the United States (U.S.) House of Representatives version of the Elder Justice Act, one of the goals is to ". . . provide for law enforcement to work hand-in-hand with health and social service agencies that have traditionally fought alone . . ." (Emanuel, 2003).

This article examines the historic, economic, political, ideological, and social movement aspects of policies promoting collaboration between APS and law enforcement and specifically, the Elder Justice Act (Blau, 2004). The analysis is challenged by the fact that such policies in the field of elder victimization are very much in their infancy. Despite this challenge, the timing of this examination provides a unique opportunity to take a cross-sectional view at a dawning policy practice. Through this perspective, those who advocate for such reform can be further enlightened as to from where elder justice policies have evolved and even perhaps where they may be headed. At the very least, this endeavor will hopefully contribute to the growing amount of material educating advocates and professionals who serve older persons about elder justice and the Elder Justice Act.

A CONCEPT OF ELDER JUSTICE

While no two experts may concur exactly on how to operationalize the concept of elder justice, one specific notion is thematic through much of the recent literature on intervention methodologies for elder victimization. Retired Louisiana Senator John Breaux (2002a) articulates this concept in his policy definition of elder justice in the Elder Justice Act. He defines elder justice as ". . . assuring that adequate public-private infrastructure and resources exist to prevent, detect, treat, understand, intervene in and, where appropriate, prosecute elder abuse, neglect, and exploitation" (p. 33). Through the proposed legislative initiatives found in the Act, his idea of elder justice, in part, involves the establishment and advancement of policies targeted toward enhancing the relationship of APS, the primary social service system charged with intervening in cases of elder victimization, and law enforcement, police, detectives, sheriffs, district attorneys, and coroners.

TYPES OF ABUSE REQUIRING LAW ENFORCEMENT AND APS COLLABORATION

The most prevalent forms of elder victimization that fall under the jurisdiction of policies utilizing relationships between APS and law enforcement are physical assault, neglect by another person, sexual abuse, and financial exploitation (Bergeron & Gray, 2003). All of these types share the common characteristic of involving a perpetrator other than the victim. Despite the fact that self-neglect is the most prevalent form of abuse referred to and substantiated by APS, there are few, if any, advocates or policy initiatives suggesting the need for the involvement of law enforcement in this clearly social service matter (Bozinovski, 2000).

Physical assault includes direct attacks where the perpetrator makes contact with the victim or propels an object or substance at the victim (Sengstock et al., 1990). Examples are slapping, kicking, punching, misusing physical or chemical restraints, and cutting with a knife. Pillemer and Moore (1990) found that 21% of nursing home staff had witnessed another staff member physically abuse a victim and 10% reported their own physically abusive behavior.

A joint investigative relationship between APS and law enforcement helped a 77-year old Pennsylvania (PA) man, after his son's home, where he resided, became a house of horror (Mattar, 2004). APS assured the victim's immediate safety by placing him in a nursing home away from the abuser. Through the collaborative relationship between the APS and law enforcement responders in this case, the son was arrested for simple assault as well as neglect of a care-dependent person, a criminal felony charge in PA. The charges stemmed from the son's physical assault that left the victim with a black right eye, cut on his forehead, large bruise on his face, and large bruise on his chest. The victim told the investigators that his son strikes out when he, the victim, urinates on himself. In his denial of the acts, the son stated, "Sure, I would throw him around–I'm rough. I'd throw him out of the bed, clean up, and then throw him back. It leaves marks and bruises on him. But if I hit him, I wouldn't be able to stop and he'd be dead" (Mattar, 2004).

Much of the literature includes sexual abuse as physical assault (Sengstock et al., 1990). For the purposes at hand, sexual abuse is separated from physical assault as it has distinct investigation and intervention methodologies. Sexual abuse is illustrated by a recent case in PA involving a 77-year-old female with Alzheimer's disease (Herman, 2004). She lived in a nursing home where a non-resident 63-year-old male sexually assaulted her. The perpetrator asked a nurse's aide to leave the room during a visit. Upon the aide's return several minutes later, she saw the perpetrator partially naked and assaulting the woman. The county where the crime occurred has a special elder abuse task force, which enables law enforcement and APS to investigate cases together. Through their joint efforts, the perpetrator plead guilty to attempted aggravated indecent assault and will no longer have the opportunity to prey upon the victim.

Sexual abuse includes any form of non-consenting sexual contact, coerced nudity, or sexually explicit photographing. Residents in long-term care settings are at increased risk to sexual predators due to many factors such as sleeping in unlocked rooms and requiring physical care from the perpetrator (Hodge, 1998). Older persons living at home are also at risk. A British study revealed that perpetrators of sexual assault against older females are mostly committed by sons (55%), son-in-laws (12%), and grandsons (12%) (Holt, 1993). Another study found that, while 80% of the perpetrators were strangers, 72% of assaults occurred in the victim's home (Muram et al., 1992). While these studies conflict on the relationship of the perpetrator, they confirm that older persons are not immune from sexual violence in their own home.

Sexual abuse is the least reported and substantiated category of victimization for APS and garners very little collaboration between APS and law enforcement. Research of referrals to the Texas APS system indicated that only 92 cases of sexual abuse were reported from a population of 2,000,000 people over the age of 65 (Pavlik et al., 2001). From 1996 to 1999, the Virginia protective services system had only 42 substantiated cases of sexual abuse for individuals over the age of 60 (Teaster et al., 2000). Only two of these cases were successfully prosecuted. APS and law enforcement conducted a joint investigation in just 14 of the cases. There is no reason to believe that these statistics do not reflect the situation throughout the U.S.

Neglect is the failure to provide the goods, care and services that are essential to the well-being of a dependent older person (Sengstock et al., 1990). Examples include being burned from water that is too hot, lack of repositioning resulting in bedsores, or strangulation through inappropriate mechanical restraints. The act of neglect can be of a criminal nature. Additionally, the subsequent actions to cover up an incident increase the likelihood of need for criminal charges and joint investigations.

A neglect case in Pittsburgh, PA involved an 88-year-old resident of an assisted living facility who suffered from Alzheimer's disease (Lash & Rotstein, 2004). She died after being left trapped outdoors in a courtyard in 40-degree temperatures. Instead of immediately reporting the incident, the supervisor on duty, upon discovery of the woman's body, ordered the body dragged back to bed. Next, the supervisor had the thermostat in the room turned up in order to reheat the body. The records were falsified to give the appearance that the victim had died of natural causes. The family was called and told that their mother had died peacefully in her sleep. After a nurse's aide at the facility reported what had happened to authorities, charges were filed. Charges in this case ranged from conspiracy to involuntary manslaughter. Due to the high profile nature of this case, the District Attorney in Allegheny County, where Pittsburgh is located, is pursuing a policy that will bring together APS and law enforcement in a task force to collaboratively intervene in cases of elder victimization.

The results of financial exploitation are no less tragic than physical assault, sexual assault or neglect. Within a short period of time, individuals can be stripped of their material possessions and independence (Choi et al., 1999; Wilber & Reynolds, 1996). Lori Stiegel in her testimony to the U.S. Senate Committee on the Judiciary on September 24, 2003, stated, "Older people may have less ability to recover from financial exploitation if they are already retired, have limited resources, or a short remaining life span." While every jurisdiction has separate names for financial crimes, this category typically involves the illegal use of funds or resources through force, misrepresentation or activities that capitalize on an older person's compromised mental state (Heisler & Tewksbury, 1991; Wilber & Reynolds, 1996).

A 58-year-old man stole nearly $200,000 utilizing a power of attorney from his 80-year-old mother to bolster his collection of Cadillac cars. He was sentenced to 18 months to three years in state prison and ordered to pay restitution of $137,809 (Young, 2003). The outcome of this case was a result of an elder abuse task force between the District Attorney and APS in Berks County, PA. Prior to the policies directing the collaborative relationship, not one case, referred from the APS unit to law enforcement in this county, had ever been successfully prosecuted, nor was any money ever recuperated for the victims.

HISTORY AND CURRENT INTERVENTIONS

The advantages, techniques and even challenges for effective collaboration will not be reviewed as they have been discussed elsewhere in the literature (Choi et al., 1999; Heisler & Tewksbury, 1991; Plotkin, 1996; Quinn & Heisler, 2002; Stiegel, 2003). It is important to recreate a policy timeline of efforts to bring together law enforcement and APS. It is also important to look at some of the more significant general elder abuse policy milestones that have affected this present concept of elder justice.

Federal Policies

Elder abuse intervention first began to receive federal recognition in the 1950s (Wolf, 2003). Public welfare officials confronted a growing population of older persons in need of services to be able to function on a day-to-day basis. A White House Conference on Aging report in 1961 stimulated the discussion regarding protective services by recommending multi-disciplinary cooperation for abuse victims. Congress also provided money to do demonstration projects. These demonstration projects began formalizing APS policies.

In 1963, Senator Frank Moss began investigating nursing home care (Anonymous, 2002). In 1965 the Older Americans Act, according to Roby and Sullivan (2000), "represented the watershed of this new awareness and activism" (p. 18). Over the next 15 years, all 50 states enacted laws to provide protective services (Daly & Jogerst, 2001; Roby & Sullivan, 2000). This process was hastened with the 1974 amendment of the Social Security Act, which mandated the institution of these services. In 1978, a congressional investigation into the problem of elder abuse was launched through the House Aging Committee which then published a report in 1981 (Roybal, 1992; Blakely & Dolon, 2000). The report brought increased national attention to the issue.

Local police departments were the primary investigators for institutional abuse in the 1970s (Hodge, 1998). This changed when, in 1977, the U.S. Senate Special Committee on Aging's Subcommittee on Long-Term Care found that Medicaid fraud was an epidemic, abuse was widespread, and prosecution by local authorities was almost nonexistent. Congress then required state level Medicaid Fraud Control Units to investigate fraud and prosecute abuse and neglect in institutional settings receiving Medicaid funds. The units receive federal and state dollars and as of 1998 had obtained 8,000 convictions for fraud and abuse.

In 1980, the Senate and House Committees on Aging held combined hearings on elder abuse (Anonymous, 2002). The Prevention, Identification, and Treatment of Adult Abuse Bill of 1981 imitated the Child Abuse Prevention and Treatment Act by seeking to federalize the response to elder abuse. Despite several attempts, the bill was never enacted. It did have the aftershock effects of encouraging states to enact mandatory reporting laws and encouraging the establishment of the National Center on Elder Abuse (NCEA) by the Administration on Aging (AoA). Also in 1980, Surgeon General Louis Sullivan began the first initiatives to bring law enforcement into the intervention system for elder abuse (Wolf, 2003). His family violence workshop, which included the issue of elder victimization, made clear that family violence was not only a public health but also a criminal justice issue.

In 1987, Congress passed further Amendments to the Older Americans Act to add a separate provision, "Elder Abuse Prevention Activities" (cited in Benoit, 1992). These amendments address elder abuse through public education, identification of abuse, and methods for receiving reports of abuse. The efforts were to be funded at $5 million in fiscal year 1988 and added to as necessary in subsequent years. These monies were never set aside (Benoit, 1992; Roybal, 1992).

The primary source of federal funding for elder abuse intervention has come through the Social Services Block Grant (Roybal, 1992). Over the 1980s, this source of funding was cut by nearly one-third due to direct cuts and inflation. In 1990, $2.9 million for elder abuse prevention was allocated for the first time (Benoit, 1992). This amount needs to be appreciated in light of the fact that it was spread over all 50 states, the District of Columbia and Territories.

In 1992, the Family Violence Prevention and Services Act was enacted (Thomas, 2000). This act enabled the Administration for Children and Families and the AoA to fund the National Elder Abuse Incidence Study (NEAIS) (Cyphers, 1999). This study examined the incidence of both reported and unreported cases of maltreatment of non-institutionalized older persons. This study is the political benchmark for data on elder victimization. It successfully advanced the Iceberg theory, which states that only the tip of the iceberg of actual cases is ever identified. The research indicates that as many as 84% of cases are never reported to APS, ombudsmen or law enforcement. Despite the positives of the NEAIS findings, advocates were concerned that the number of victims did not meet a political threshold to convince legislators of the need for federal action (Thomas, 2000).

A piece of federal legislation for victims of all ages impacted service to older crime victims. The Victims of Crime Act Fund, passed in 1984, helps victims of crime by reimbursing the individual for damages from the crime (Deem, 2000). To qualify for the assistance, victims must press charges against the perpetrator. Victims can be reimbursed for such items as medical expenses, counseling, and lost wages. Until 1997, victims of financial crimes were not able to access assistance through this fund. Today, financial crimes victims are now considered underserved and are given priority for funding. This Act pointed out the necessity for responses to meet both the justice and service needs of victims.

Most recently, Senators John Breaux of Louisiana, a Democrat, and Orrin Hatch of Utah, a Republican, introduced the Elder Justice Act on September 13, 2002. The Act was reintroduced in the 108th Congressional session as S. 333 (Stiegel, 2004). It had a companion bill in the House, H.R. 2490. The Act's goals include funding and promoting relationships between APS and law enforcement (Breaux, 2002b). At the time of completing this article, the Act has not reached the floor of the House or Senate for a vote despite bipartisan support.

State Policies

While federal policy has been lacking, states have taken steps to move toward the goal of developing law enforcement and APS responses to elder victimization. State legislative efforts differ by jurisdictions. States such as California have a separate section of the penal code dedicated to the abuse of older persons and dependent adults (Allen, 2000). Other states have no separate legislation for older adults, instead utilizing their general crimes code. California passed legislation in 2001 allowing counties to establish death review teams to review elder abuse and neglect cases (Dayton, 2002). These teams are made up of law enforcement and APS as well as other professionals.

State Attorney Generals have been at the forefront of blending law enforcement with APS efforts. The Florida Attorney General's Office created "Operation Spot Check" which conducts unannounced inspections of institutions in Broward and Palm Beach counties with a team of inspectors that include law enforcement as well as APS (Hodge, 1998). The goal of the team is to prevent problems by doing thorough inspections of the facilities from a multi-disciplinary perspective.

Oregon's Attorney General created an elder abuse task force in 1994 including law enforcement and APS (Kaye & Darling, 2000). From the efforts of this task force, initiatives grew to educate bank employees about how to recognize financial crime being perpetrated against older persons. The task force also taught seniors to understand that certain telemarketing and mail marketing schemes are crimes and should be reported to the authorities.

Community Policies

Within the states, municipalities have adopted policies to address elder victimization in their communities through law enforcement and APS relationships. The Los Angeles Police Department established the Elder Person's Estate Unit and the Los Angles County Area Agency on Aging established the Fiduciary Abuse Specialist Team (FAST) to specifically target elder financial exploitation (Aziz, 2000; Deem, 2000). These programs were two of the first to formally bring together law enforcement and APS as well as other disciplines to respond to cases. FAST type teams were also established for Orange and Contra Costa Counties in California, Santa Clara, California, Dane County, Wisconsin, and King County, Washington (Allen, 2000).

Another effort originating out of California involves social services working with the FBI and the U.S. Postal Inspectors as well as other agencies to establish the National Telemarketing Victim Call Center for seniors in Los Angeles County (Aziz et al., 2000). This program allows authorities to work collaboratively to be responsive to telemarketing scams, which are very difficult to investigate and resolve.

Multi-disciplinary teams, which include APS and law enforcement, have sprung up across the country. In Reading, PA, police, District Attorney, APS, domestic violence, sexual assault, coroner, and victims' compensation representatives meet every six weeks to discuss cases. During the year and a half of meetings, they have made over 15 arrests allowing them to both deliver service and obtain justice for the victims. The Pennsylvania Commission on Crime and Delinquency and Temple University's Institute on Protective Services are working to establish task forces in other Pennsylvania counties.

The Brevard County prosecutor's office in Florida is using formalized investigative relationships to combat elder victimization (Miller & Johnson, 2003). A protocol was established between APS and law enforcement that delineates the responsibilities and procedures for an investigation when criminality is suspected in a case of abuse, neglect or exploitation. Despite these examples of successful policy initiatives on the local level, a recent survey of local prosecutors found only a few utilizing interagency teams in responding to crimes against older persons.

IDEOLOGY

Several different ideological debates exist when discussing collaboration between law enforcement and APS. The first debate is over the question of why perpetrators victimize older persons. The caregiver stress model suggests that perpetrators are well meaning but at increased risk to victimizing due to the difficulties and challenges of care giving (Bergeron & Gray, 2003; Brandl, 2000). This model was the prevalent view in the late 1970s and through the 1980s, thus providing much of the theoretical foundation for existing APS laws and policies.

Those who look at abuse from a caregiver stress model tend to favor, as the primary intervention, social service methods that attempt to relieve stress and make the care-giving situation successful. In 1988, Dr. Callahan, Jr. (2000) argued,

> First, these abuse problems should be considered, in most cases, as falling within the domain of the social service system. The knowledge (limited though it may be) and skilled motivated staff exist within this system. A broad social service approach [including mental health] should be undertaken to meet the varied needs of older persons. To divert needed resources into criminalizing social problems or to thoughtlessly reallocate them from within a starved social service system to special abuse program will be disastrous. (p. 35)

In fairness to Dr. Callahan, he does later acknowledge that where crimes are broken, crimes should be enforced but the emphasis on the ideology that the social service system should be the primary player in confronting abuse is abundant in current protective services policy and practice.

Other experts do not see abuse as due to caregiver stress but have suggested other models that place the emphasis upon the perpetrator by describing characteristics of perpetrators that have little to do with stress. This mindset implies that people, who do not have predisposed characteristics that make them vulnerable to victimizing, find other healthy mechanisms to deal with the burdens of care giving. Those who look at models that focus on the perpetrator such as the family violence model and perpetrator dependency theory are more in favor of utilizing both APS and law enforcement as part of the intervention. These theorists argue that when professionals legitimize stress as a reason for victimization, interventions are rarely effective and in some cases even increase the risk to the victim (Brandl, 2000). The arrest and, at times, imprisonment sends the message to the perpetrator as well as the community that victimization of older persons is not only inappropriate but also illegal.

The Right of Self-Determination

Another ideological debate in this discussion of elder justice is whether elder crime is against the person or the person and community. This is brought into the practical world in the debate as to whether a victim has the right to self-determination in reporting a crime to law enforcement and pressing criminal charges against the perpetrator, or whether criminal prosecution should proceed if sufficient evidence exists regardless of the will of the victim. Rosalie Wolf (1996) stated:

> Certainly, the refusal of the victim to press charges has been a major barrier to intervention efforts. Even though the law may require an investigation, the older person may not wish to cooperate or to accept the services that are offered. This negative response brings the worker face to face with a dilemma: the interest of the state and professional practice in protecting vulnerable persons and the individual's right to self-determination. (p. 88)

While most of the APS literature supports the client's right to self-determination in reporting to police and filing criminal charges, the ideological debate has existed since the idea of APS and law enforcement becoming partners in intervention started (Heisler & Tewksbury, 1991). During the 1990 APS Conference in San Antonio, a case example regarding multi-disciplinary issues was discussed (Mixson et al., 1992). During the discussion, this ideological debate arose. Candace Heisler, JD, articulated the view that does not absolutely defer to the right of self-determination when deciding whether to proceed with prosecution. When asked if the prosecutor needs the victim's permission to press charges, she responded:

> Speaking generally of the law: No prosecutor must ask a victim if he or she is interested in prosecution. When do you suppose was the last time a murder victim was asked if he or she wanted a prosecution? We charge whether or not the victim is available, on the basis of our responsibility to protect society and to recognize our role as the attorney for the people that we serve ... I am the lawyer for the people of my jurisdiction ... and there is a public desire that we protect the members of our community. So if you are being told in your community that victims have to prosecute, that is really a shorthand way for law enforcement and prosecution to say, 'Here's an easy way out.' We do not ask burglary victims if they want to prosecute, and in San Francisco we do not ask victims of domestic violence and elder abuse if they want to prosecute. We decide whether the evidence available to us is sufficient to support the charge. (pp. 49-50)

The opposing view was more succinctly but not less subtly expressed by Prasad Sripada, MD, who stated, "Society has the duty to protect, but the individual has the right to autonomy" (p. 50). Dessin (2000) in a separate article finds a middle ground:

In addition to personal autonomy concerns, there is a societal interest in preventing and remedying financial abuse of the elderly. It is reasonable to conclude that society should prevent, remedy, or punish financial abuse, or perhaps do all three. This concern may be strong enough to overcome certain aspects of personal autonomy, but such paternalism should not be undertaken without good reason.

Federalism

Finally, policies on elder victimization have developed during a time of the conservative ideology of federalism (Teaster & Anetzberger, 2002). Teaster and Anetzberger assert:

> Unlike child abuse, the federal government did not provide the states with policy direction and incentives. An even more conservative approach made elder abuse a family or personal problem, with responsibility for resolution up to the individuals most affected rather than a broader one with responsibilities at multiple levels of the individual, the family, the community, and the state. (p. xv)

The Elder Justice Act was crafted in order to try and avoid this issue (Elder Justice Coalition, 2004). The legislation avoids federalizing the local response to elder victimization but instead attempts to offer federal leadership and resources. The Elder Justice Coalition's web site states:

> This is a 'smart' bill. The goal is to create a minimal federal infrastructure to efficiently address elder abuse as the problem grows, especially with the aging of the boomers. It tries to take a more progressive approach to this national problem, by putting prevention at the heart of the effort, using private and public resources, and providing federal leadership to help empower local communities to care for their own.

POLITICS

Congressman Edward R. Roybal stated in 1992 that:

> . . . present-day America is an 'eleventh hour' nation, which musters its political will and seeks solutions to its problems only in the presence of a crisis . . . In the area of adult abuse, neglect, and exploitation, we are already in a crisis. And the crisis is of such magnitude that it impels us all, politicians, social workers, concerned neighbors, and family members, and elders themselves, to work for change. (p. 64)

Over 10 years later the Elder Justice Act has achieved some political success. As of June, 2004, it had bipartisan support with 42 cosponsors in the senate and 82 cosponsors in the House as of March, 2004 (Fuller, 2004).

Unfortunately, Senator Breaux, the champion of the Elder Justice Act, retired. The departure of such a strong advocate for this legislation leaves the bill's fate hanging delicately in the balance (Stiegel, 2004). One of the legislative roadblocks had been Senator Larry Craig, Republican from Idaho, who is the chairman of the Senate Special Committee on Aging. He had been concerned that there is not enough in the Act on guardianship misuse and about the overall cost of the bill. As of April 22nd, 2004, Senator Larry Craig joined the bipartisan list of supporters. Craig is also a member of the Appropriations Committee which could prove crucial to the adequate funding of the Act.

When asked in the frequently asked questions section of the Elder Justice Coalition web site as to who opposes the Act, they respond:

> We are currently unaware of anyone or any group who opposes the need to protect our revered senior citizens from abuse. The number and breadth of organizations and interest groups that are represented in the Elder Justice Coalition who all favor the Elder Justice Proposal is an example of how well this bill has been received . . . We recognize that 'devil is in the details' and that many will have specific interests. However, it is our hope that we can keep our 'eye on the ball' and pass this desperately needed legislation where Congress has been remiss for far too long. (2004)

The most powerful potential foe is the long-term care industry that does not embrace further regulation and supervision by agencies with the ability to sanction. While this industry may not take on the Elder Justice Act directly, a likely strategy will be to oppose certain parts and use those parts to kill the entire bill. To ward off this opposition, the Act, in its original version, offered several perks around the issue of staffing, a major issue in long-term care. Grants and tax incentives were included to recruit and retain long-term care workers.

To date many of the political battles over law enforcement and APS relationships have been fought on the local level. District Attorneys are elected politicians. District attorneys are a key building stone to implementing policies that utilize relationships between the law enforcement community and APS (Miller & Johnson, 2003). As the chief local law enforcement officer, their involvement or lack thereof sets the precedent for the community. Unfortunately, in many jurisdictions their level of interest or at least the perception of their level of interest in elder victimization is low. In a study by Blakely and

Dolon (2000), APS workers reported prosecution as a top service to address elder abuse but ranked it as difficult to achieve. APS workers and elder victimization advocates find low level of prosecutor interest to be a significant barrier to achieving prosecution.

Elder victimization advocates must be aware, when advocating to District Attorneys, that this issue competes with other high profile crimes such as drugs, street violence and drinking and driving. As will be discussed under social movements, media coverage and high profile cases can be utilized by advocates to convince District Attorneys of the need for and political benefits of collaborative relationships on this issue.

In 2001, the NCEA national action agenda considered a political strategy of pursuing an Executive Order by the President to implement the review of elder abuse services. The NCEA proceedings to develop the agenda were held from December 4th to 6th, 2001. While not discussed, perhaps the members of the work groups thought that homeland security would not continue to demand the attention that it has. Nevertheless given the current Iraq war and the concerns regarding homeland security, neither the President nor the Congress have shown significant public interest in this issue.

SOCIAL MOVEMENTS

Social movements around elder justice have simply not happened in any organized manner. It can be argued that no social movement has existed specific to elder abuse but that success in elder abuse policy has only coat tailed on the movements of child abuse and domestic violence. While social movements have not existed, there have been peaks of interest. In the 1970s, a series of events peaked interest including an episode of the popular television show, Quincy, M.E., detailing a medical examiner's look at a case of elder abuse (Payne & Berg, 2003). The term "granny battering" originated in England and became an international catch phrase to help bring the issue to public recognition. In both the 1980s and 1990s, experts picked each of those decades to be the one when elder abuse would be pushed forward by a major social movement (Payne et al., 1999). While these decades did allow elder abuse to blip on the national radar, the idea of elder justice was still off the screen.

These peaks of interest about elder abuse allowed for the implementation of policies that have set the stage for elder justice today. For example, mandatory reporting laws and special sentencing guidelines were enacted in many jurisdictions as a step to increase prosecutions (Payne et al., 2001). But as far as a social movement toward elder justice, the 1980s and 1990s and even the early 2000s have passed with little to show.

Within aging, many social movements live and die by the involvement or lack thereof of one organization, the American Association of Retired Persons (AARP). Rosalie Wolf said, "The elder's voice has been absent from the discourse on elder abuse . . . The topic has been defined and promoted only by professionals" (cited in Heller, 2002, p. 63). If the AARP is any part of the seniors' voices, it has been seemingly silent. In 1992, Richard L. Douglass wrote that:

> The American Association of Retired Persons . . . has been in the vanguard of national efforts to bring domestic mistreatment of the elderly to the consciousness of the general public since the issue came to public attention in 1978 . . . Unlike many sustained efforts, however, the AARP emphasis has been on prevention and the empowerment of the elderly to anticipate risk and to prepare for their aging in ways that might minimize the probability of being victims of neglectful or abusive treatment. (p. 74)

Years later this still seems to be the stance of the AARP (NCEA, 2001). Additionally, AARP has let state chapters decide their level of interest on the issue. State AARP chapters have been active in elder abuse and elder justice legislation in states such as Utah, Maryland, Kentucky, New York, and Iowa. In New York, the AARP chapter dealt with APS and law enforcement collaboration in its support and assistance to the State's TRIAD program (Heller, 2002). While in 2002, AARP did have a representative at the introduction of the Elder Justice Act, the stance of the AARP on this issue has done little to advance a social movement for change.

In 2001, the NCEA, an organization made up of six partner agencies, decided to formulate a public policy action agenda. Their goals were on the mark to create a social movement. They included developing a national policy agenda for domestic and institutional abuse, raising awareness about the issues, promoting interdisciplinary involvement, and establishing a task force to advance the agenda. Furthermore, the goals of these efforts included filling service gaps, enhancing APS, increasing prosecution, and maximizing resources. This was applied to APS and law enforcement collaboration policy in their idea to increase awareness within the justice system:

> Elder abuse and neglect must become a priority crime control issue. The justice system including law enforcement, prosecution, corrections, judiciary, medical examiners/coroners, public safety officers, victim advocates, APS workers, Ombudsmen, and others must work as a coordinated system to: Protect victims; Hold offenders accountable; Prevent future offenses. (p. 4)

The level of interest in elder victimization and the concept of elder justice is arguably at an all time high (Stiegel, 2004). The Elder Justice Coalition has been formed to build a social movement. It currently has over 300 individual and organizational members. Its web site, www.elderjusticecoalition.com, contains tools for advocates including letters to senators, information, and talking points.

A current concern is whether elder justice has generated enough interest and activity beyond academicians and a small group of advocates, specifically victims and frontline professionals. When examining the history of social movements such as domestic violence, it was when victims became engaged along with advocates that great strides were gained (Payne et al., 2001). Due to the physical and cognitive limitations of older victims, the ability to mobilize action among this population is hindered.

Thus, it is imperative that the frontline APS worker be engaged in a social movement. Marshall Pierson (2003), an APS worker from Ohio, believes that satisfaction from achieving successful outcomes for victims through collaboration with law enforcement not only benefits the victim but also has a strong benefit to APS. Many in the APS system agree with this idea but are not active because they perceive it as too utopian, something that will never happen in the real world. Pierson writes "The seven most deadly words to prevent change are: 'We've never done it that way before.' Precisely. And that's why we continue to see the same dismal, demoralizing outcomes" (p. 67).

Social movements require buzzwords with clear definitions. This has not been the case with elder justice or even elder abuse. Much of the literature laments the lack of clear definitions for abuse and neglect (Payne et al., 1999). A definition is important in setting the goals to be sought by a social movement. Payne et al. point out:

> Though a definition is missing in the literature, or perhaps because a definition is missing, research concurs that a consistent definition among legislatures, academicians, practitioners, criminal justice officials, and the elderly is needed in order to effectively detect, intervene, and prevent elder abuse. (p. 63)

Social movements are also dependent on media coverage. The NCEA recognized this when listing educating the media as a key point to public recognition of the issue (2001). After an undercover investigation of a chain of nursing homes in PA, the media became instrumental in building a social movement (Costen, 1996). Due to the grizzly pictures of individuals literally rotting to death, the television, radio and print media outlets became interested in the story. Advocates and the public became outraged and called upon the

PA General Assembly to act in order to ensure a minimum level of care in nursing homes. Despite intense pressure from the nursing home industry to defeat the legislation, the social movement was too great and the Care Dependent Mistreatment Act was passed.

More recently in PA, the case of an 83-year-old man who was stomped by a night attendant in a personal-care home and then left to suffer for six days until he died appalled the Bucks County District Attorney so much that she aggressively pursued prosecution and succeeded (King, 2004). Additionally, a significant degree of media attention followed the case which created public outrage. The District Attorney, emboldened by the media coverage and public reaction, has formed a task force between law enforcement and APS to better intervene in elder victimization cases.

ECONOMICS

In 1985, Representative Claude Pepper issued a report that indicated that states spent $22.14 per child for protective services but only $2.91 for older persons (Anonymous, 2002). In 1990, the Subcommittee on Health and Long-Term Care of the House Select Committee on Aging found $45.03 was spent for children and $3.80 for older persons. Currently, 153.5 million federal dollars go to elder abuse, only 2% of the federal spending for all forms of abuse (Fuller, 2004).

At this time, only Title VII (Vulnerable Elder Rights Protection Activities) of the Older Americans Act provides funding, which is targeted to elder abuse. The majority of states (32) utilize the Social Services Block Grant to fund APS and elder abuse efforts (NCEA, 2001). The Social Services Block Grant has been victim to many cuts over the years (Anonymous, 2002). It also does not specifically earmark monies for protective services for older persons. APS units claim their biggest problem to be lack of funding and face budget issues so dire that they risk not being able to serve clients, let alone to pursue elder justice (Mixson, 2002; Otto & Bell, 2003).

Unfortunately, research has not been done as to the taxpayer cost of elder victimization (Stiegel, 2003). Costs may include hospitalization or nursing home placement. When individuals lose their assets, their dependence on public assistance grows. Such public subsidies include cash assistance, housing, and Medical Assistance for long-term care.

The Elder Justice Act started at an estimated cost of $650 million per year for the seven years of the bill (Elder Justice Coalition, 2004). As of June, 2004, the amount being discussed in the capital is down to less than $300 million per year (Fuller, 2004). Either of these amounts may seem costly but are only a fraction of the cost spent on other types of abuse. Child abuse receives $7 billion in federal funding annually. Just the needed resources to compile a national reporting system will require a large federal appropriation, let alone what all of the other elements of the Act will need (Goodrich, 1997).

Economics will remain a key issue to the success or failure of the Elder Justice Act and efforts to build collaborative relationships between law enforcement and APS. The money will come when enough people are outraged by the failures of both law enforcement and APS to handle these cases separately. The media is starting to scrutinize the existing system and are finding the lack of collaboration unpalatable (Cook-Daniels, 2004). Unfortunately when depending on political funding, the problem sometimes needs to get worse before it gets better.

CONCLUSION

Some may argue that law enforcement and APS collaboration is not a significant social work policy issue. The scattered but consistent successful results form such policies across the U.S. prove otherwise. The Elder Justice Act provides an unprecedented opportunity to create, enhance and standardize relationships between APS and law enforcement through the leadership of federal policy. While the ideological fights rage, while the politics are negotiated, while the economics are haggled and while the social movement is ignited, millions of older persons face the reality of victimization and a system whose response provides only part of their needs, at best. It is only when there is collaboration between APS and law enforcement that elder justice can be obtained. When part of the policies of elder justice include collaboration between APS and law enforcement, victims gain safety, restoration and peace of mind, a very worthy policy goal indeed.

REFERENCES

Allen, J. V. (2000). Financial abuse of elders and dependent adults: The FAST (Financial Abuse Specialist Team). *Journal of Elder Abuse & Neglect*, 12(2), 85-92.

Anonymous (2002). Protecting older Americans: A history of federal action on elder abuse, neglect, and exploitation. *Journal of Elder Abuse & Neglect*, 14(2/3), 9-30.

Aziz, S.J. (2000). Los Angeles county fiduciary abuse specialist team: A model for collaboration. *Journal of Elder Abuse & Neglect*, 12(2), 79-84.

Aziz, S.J., Bolick, D.C., Kleinman, M.T., & Shadel, D.P. (2000). The national telemarketing victim call center: Combating telemarketing fraud in the United States. *Journal of Elder Abuse & Neglect*, 12(2), 93-98.

Benoit, M.D. (1992). Elder abuse: A legislative update. *Journal of Elder Abuse & Neglect*, 3(4), 63-71.

Bergeron, L.R., & Gray, B. (2003). Ethical dilemmas of reporting suspected elder abuse. *Social Work*, 48(1), 96-105.

Blakely, B.E., & Dolon, R. (2000). Perceptions of adult protective services workers of the support provided by criminal justice professionals in a case of elder abuse. *Journal of Elder Abuse & Neglect*, 12(3/4), 71-92.

Blau, J. (2004). *The dynamics of social welfare policy*. New York: Oxford University Press.

Bozinovski, S.D. (2000). Older self-neglecters: Interpersonal problems and the maintenance of self-continuity. *Journal of Elder Abuse & Neglect*, 12(1), 37-56.

Brandl, B. (2000). Power and control: Understanding domestic abuse in later life. *Generations*, 24(2), 39-45.

Breaux, J. (2002a). S 333 IS–108th Congress, 1st session: To promote elder justice, and for other purposes. *Journal of Elder Abuse & Neglect*, 14(2/3), 87-189.

Breaux, J. (2002b). Senator Breaux's elder justice proposal of 2002 executive summary. *Journal of Elder Abuse & Neglect*, 14(2/3), 33-36.

Callahan, J.J. (2000). Elder abuse revisited. *Journal of Elder Abuse & Neglect*, 12(1), 33-37.

Choi, N.G., Kulick, D. B., & Mayer, J. (1999). Financial exploitation of elders: Analysis of risk factors based on county adult protective services data. *Journal of Elder Abuse & Neglect*, 10(3/4), 39-61.

Cook-Daniels, L. (2004). Florida's elder abuse system comes under fire. *Victimization of the Elderly & Disabled*, 6(6), 87 & 90.

Costen, R.W. (1996). The criminal prosecutor's roles in assuring quality of care in long term care settings. *Journal of Elder Abuse & Neglect*, 8(3), 21-36.

Cyphers, G. C. (1999). Elder abuse and neglect. *Policy & Practice of Public Human Services*, 57(3), 25-30.

Daly, J., & Jogerst, G. (2001). Statute definitions of elder abuse. *Journal of Elder Abuse & Neglect*, 13(4), 39-57.

Dayton, K. (2002). Legislative roundup–New state laws protecting vulnerable adults. *Victimization of the Elderly and Disabled*, 5(4), 53-54.

Deem, D. (2000). Notes from the field: Observations in working with forgotten victims of personal financial crimes. *Journal of Elder Abuse & Neglect*, 12(2), 33-48.

Dessin, C.L. (2000). Financial abuse of the elderly. *Idaho Law Review*, 36(203). Retrieved June 23, 2004 from LexisNexis.™

Douglass, R. (1992). Reaching 30 million people to prevent abuse and neglect of the elderly: AARP's strategy for public self-education. *Journal of Elder Abuse & Neglect*, 3(4), 73-85.

Elder Justice Coalition's questions and answers page (n.d.). Retrieved May 10, 2004 from http://www.elderjusticecoalition.org/q_a.htm

Emanuel, R. (2003). *Emanuel introduces elder justice act*. Retrieved June 1, 2004 from http://www.house.gov/apps/list/press/il05_emanuel/Elder_Justice_Act.html

Fuller, L. (2004, June). Protecting our greatest generation: The view from the hill. In *National Symposium on Financial Exploitation and Abuse*. Washington, DC.

Goodrich, C. S. (1997). Results of a national survey of state protective services programs: Assessing risk and defining victim outcomes. *Journal of Elder Abuse & Neglect*, 9(1), 69-86.

Heisler, C.J., & Tewksbury, J.E. (1991). Fiduciary abuse of the elderly: A prosecutor's perspective. *Journal of Elder Abuse & Neglect*, 3(4), 23-40.

Heller, J. (2002). Where is AARP regarding elder abuse? *Victimization of the Elderly and Disabled*, 5(4), 49 & 63.

Herman, H. (2003, March 28). Man, 63, pleads guilty to attempted sexual assault. *Reading Eagle*.

Hodge, P.D. (1998). National law enforcement programs to prevent, detect, investigate, and prosecute elder abuse and neglect in health care facilities. *Journal of Elder Abuse & Neglect*, 9(4), 23-41.

Holt, M.G. (1993). Elder sexual abuse in Britain: Preliminary findings. *Journal of Elder Abuse & Neglect*, 5(2), 63-71.

Kaye, A., & Darling, G. (2000). Oregon's efforts to reduce elder financial exploitation. *Journal of Elder Abuse & Neglect*, 12(2), 99-102.

King, L. (2004, May 26). From tragedy, positive steps to safeguard elders. *The Philadelphia Inquirer*. Retrieved June 3, 2004 from http://www.philly.com/mld/inquirer/news/local/states/pennsylvania/8759245.htm?1c

Lash, C., & Rostein, G. (2003, October 23). Nursing home charged. *Post-gazette.com*. Retrieved October 28, 2003 from http://www.post-gazette.com/printer.asp

Mattar, G. (2004, March 26). Man charged with abusing elderly dad. *Phillyburbs.com*. Retrieved March 29, 2004 from http://www.phillyburbs.com/pb-dyn/articlePrint.cfm?id=271524

Miller, M.L., & Johnson, J.L. (2003). *Protecting America's senior citizens: What local prosecutors are doing to fight elder abuse*. Alexandria, VA: American Prosecutors Research Institute.

Mixson, P.M. (2002). Taking a leap forward: Adult protective services and the elder justice act. *Journal of Elder Abuse & Neglect*, 14(2/3), 193-197.

Mixson, P., Chelucci, K., Heisler, C., Overman, W., Sripada, P., & Yates, P. (1992). The case of Mrs. M.–A multidisciplinary team staffing. *Journal of Elder Abuse & Neglect*, 3(4), 41-55.

Muram, D., Miller, K., & Cutler, A. (1992). Sexual assault of the elderly victim. *Journal of Interpersonal Violence*, 7(1), 70-76.

National Center on Elder Abuse (2001). *The national policy summit on elder abuse: Creating the action agenda*.

Otto, J., & Bell, J.C. (2003). *Problems facing state adult protective services programs and the resources needed to resolve them*. Denver: National Association of Adult Protective Services Administrators.

Pavlik, V.N., Hyman, D.J., Festa, N. A., & Dyer, C. B. (2001). Quantifying the problem of abuse and neglect in adults–Analysis of a statewide database. *Journal of the American Geriatrics Society*, 49(1), 45-48.

Payne, B.K., Berg, B.L., & Byars, K. (1999). A qualitative examination of the similarities and differences of elder abuse definitions among four groups: Nursing home directors, nursing home employees, police chiefs and students. *Journal of Elder Abuse & Neglect*, 10(3/4), 63-85.

Payne, B.K., Berg, B.L., & Toussaint, J. (2001). The police response to the criminalization of elder abuse: An exploratory study. *Policing*, 24(4), 605-625.

Payne, B. K., & Berg, B. (2003). Perceptions about the criminalization of elder abuse among police chiefs and ombudsmen. *Crime & Delinquency*, 49(3), 439-459.

Pierson, M. (2003). Autobiography of one adult protective services practitioner in a transitional small Midwestern county setting. *Victimization of the Elderly and Disabled*, 6(4), 49 & 60-62.

Pillemer, K., & Moore, D.W. (1990). Highlights from a study of abuse of patients in nursing homes. *Journal of Elder Abuse & Neglect*, 2(1/2), 5-29.

Plotkin, M.R. (1996). Improving the police response to domestic elder abuse victims. *Aging*, 367, 28.

Quinn, M.J., & Heisler, C.J. (2002). The legal system: Civil and criminal responses to elder abuse and neglect. *The Public Policy and Aging Report*, 12(2), 8-14.

Roby, J.L., & Sullivan, R. (2000). Adult protection service laws: A comparison of state statutes from definition to case closure. *Journal of Elder Abuse & Neglect*, 12(3/4), 17-52.

Roybal, E.R. (1992). Elder abuse: We must press on for increased federal support. *Journal of Elder Abuse & Neglect*, 3(4), 57-64.

Sengstock, M.C., McFarland, M.R., & Hwalek, M. (1990). Identification of elder abuse in institutional settings: Required changes in existing protocols. *Journal of Elder Abuse & Neglect*, 2(1/2), 31-50.

Stiegel, L. (2003). *Elder abuse, neglect, and exploitation: Are we doing enough?* Retrieved June 3, 2004 from http://judiciary.senate.gov/print_testimony.cfm?id=935& wit_id=2651

Stiegel, L. (2004). Washington Report. *Victimization of the Elderly and Disabled*, 6(6), 85-86 & 92.

Teaster, P.B., Roberto, K.A., Duke, J.O., & Kim, M. (2000). Sexual abuse of older adults: Preliminary findings of cases in Virginia. *Journal of Elder Abuse & Neglect*, 12(3/4), 1-16.

Teaster, P. B., & Anetzberger, G. J. (2002). Preface. *Journal of Elder Abuse & Neglect*, 14(2/3), xv-xviii.

Thomas, C. (2000). The first national study of elder abuse and neglect: Contrast with results from other studies. *Journal of Elder Abuse & Neglect*, 12(1), 1-14.

Wilber, K.H., & Reynolds, S. L. (1996). Introducing a framework for defining financial abuse of the elderly. *Journal of Elder Abuse & Neglect*, 8(2), 61-80.

Wolf, R.S. (1996). Elder abuse and family violence: Testimony presented before the U.S. senate special committee on aging. *Journal of Elder Abuse & Neglect*, 8(1), 81-96.

Wolf, R. (2003). Elder abuse and neglect: History and concepts. In R. Bonnie and R. Wallace (Eds.), *Elder mistreatment: Abuse, Neglect, and Exploitation in an Aging America* (pp. 238-248). Washington, DC: The National Academies Press.

Young, M.E. (2003, November 21). Pennside man sentenced for $200,000 theft from his mother. *Reading Eagle*.

Social Inclusion:
An Interplay of the Determinants of Health–
New Insights into Elder Abuse

Dr. Elizabeth Podnieks, EdD

SUMMARY. Social and economic exclusion and inclusion are receiving growing attention and study in North America for their usefulness as a conceptual framework that addresses the many dimensions of poverty and inequality in our society. A discussion of social and economic exclusion/inclusion flows naturally out of the population health field in which the social determinants of health have become well-established over the last twenty years or more. The determinants of health provide a broad and inclusive outline within which to situate prevention, early detection and effective intervention of the abuse of older persons. A *Social Inclusion Lens* offers exciting possibilities for addressing the issue of elder abuse and neglect. *[Article copies available for a fee from The Haworth Document Delivery Service: 1-800-HAWORTH. E-mail address: <docdelivery@haworthpress. com> Website: <http://www.HaworthPress.com> © 2006 by The Haworth Press, Inc. All rights reserved.]*

KEYWORDS. Social inclusion, elder abuse, health determinants, intervention

Appreciation is expressed to Malcolm Shookner for permission to reprint "The Inclusion Lens: Workbook for Looking at Social and Economic Exclusion and Inclusion" and to Stephanie Speer, RN, for assistance in the development of this paper.

[Haworth co-indexing entry note]: "Social Inclusion: An Interplay of the Determinants of Health–New Insights into Elder Abuse." Podnieks, Elizabeth. Co-published simultaneously in *Journal of Gerontological Social Work* (The Haworth Press, Inc.) Vol. 46, No. 3/4, 2006, pp. 57-79 ; and: *Elder Abuse and Mistreatment: Policy, Practice, and Research* (ed: M. Joanna Mellor, and Patricia Brownell) The Haworth Press, Inc., 2006, pp. 57-79. Single or multiple copies of this article are available for a fee from The Haworth Document Delivery Service [1-800-HAWORTH, 9:00 a.m. - 5:00 p.m. (EST). E-mail address: docdelivery@ haworthpress.com].

57

INTRODUCTION

Social Inclusion is . . .

> both a goal and a process. It welcomes individuals and groups who have
> been left out into the planning, decision-making, and policy-develop-
> ment processes in their community. And it empowers them by offering
> the opportunities, resource, and support they need to participate.

–Maritime Centre of Excellence for Women's Health, Dalhousie University

The word "inclusion" resonates with most of us. One of the basic needs developed by Maslow is "belonging" (Maslow, 1970). We all need to feel included, accepted, to feel we are able to participate fully within our families,
our communities, and our society. People may be excluded because of poverty, gender, race, health, lack of education, or age and consequently they do
not have the chance for full participation in the economic and social benefits of
our society. Simply put, "exclusion is the problem: inclusion is the solution"
(Guildford, 2000). Prime Minister Tony Blair offers the following definition:
"Social exclusion is about income but is about more. It is about prospects and
networks and life-chances. It's a very modern problem, and one that is more
harmful to the individual, more damaging to self-esteem, more corrosive for
society as a whole, more likely to be passed down from generation to generation than material poverty" (cited in Guildford, 2000).

The social exclusion of older adults is well documented (Brownell, 2003).
Exclusion of older people is a product of structural inequalities (Neysmith and
Edwardh, 1984). The International Plan of Action on Ageing 2002 seeks to address the social exclusion of older adults on a global scale and calls for initiatives to respond to the inequalities, marginalization, deprivation, and violence
that many older adults experience in their families and communities. Lack of
power and status makes it difficult for older people to access services; find out
and negotiate what is due to them; respond to abuse and neglect; seek accessible information; and protest against age and gender-related discrimination
(HelpAge International, 2000).

Social exclusion is most damaging when older people lack health and material support services, when they face discrimination from family and state and
when socio-economic and cultural change is very rapid and profound. Scarce
resources, isolation and physical weakness are all elements of multi-dimen-
sional disadvantages to which older people are vulnerable. These disadvantages are related to processes and institutional arrangements and deny them

full participation in the economic, social, and political life of their communities (de Haan, 1998).

The social exclusion of poor older people is closely allied to negative social and personal attitudes that construe ageing as a state of diminished capacities. Age-based prejudice isolates older people from consultation and decision-making processes at family, community, and national levels and can lead to denial of services and support on grounds of age (HelpAge International, 2000). The interplay of these circumstances can easily lead to abusive situations.

Social inclusion has been a central concept for the development of social policy in Europe for over a decade, and it is now earning support and respect in Canada. It offers a fresh way of bringing new approaches and new people to the social policy process. It has won the support of a wide variety of governments and organizations, led to the adoption of effective programs in Europe, and proven itself adaptable to a variety of cultural contexts. The value of the concept is that it recognizes that exclusion from society happens to people as a result of societal change and governance policy rather than a direction freely chosen by individuals. The processes contributing to social exclusion include economic change, changes to welfare programs, exclusion from societal participation and demographic changes such as an ageing population. Government policies serve in either increasing or decreasing the extent of social exclusion within a society (Guildford, 2000).

The language of social inclusion is making in-roads into policy debates. Health Canada's commitment to population health places it in a strategic position to bring many groups together to combat social and economic exclusion. Health Canada is the federal agency responsible for helping the people of Canada maintain and improve their health. The next step in Canada is to bring effective leadership to the process. Health Canada is well positioned to take up that challenge (Guildford, 2000). This paper encourages human service providers to develop a common understanding of social inclusion that would enable each sector to develop their own set of strategies for building inclusive communities that would protect vulnerable older people from abuse and neglect.

THE DETERMINANTS OF HEALTH

A discussion of social and economic exclusion/inclusion flows naturally out of population health field, the social determinants of which have become well established over the last twenty years or more. The determinants of health provide a broad and inclusive framework within which to situate prevention, early detection and effective intervention of the abuse of older persons. Understanding abuse and neglect of older persons will help in the design of policies and programs that work. Not only will a determinants of health approach result in preventing such situations from occurring but also will aid in the identification of those older persons who are vulnerable and at risk. Such an approach will result in early screening so that appropriate strategies may be put in place to deal with, and prevent abuse from occurring (Podnieks, 1997). The risk factors that have been summarized from diverse studies on the abuse and neglect of older persons have proven that a complex interaction among socio-economic, psychological, and environmental conditions potentially impact on the abused and the abuser. Thus, it is relevant and helpful to examine how each determinant is related to the abuse and neglect of older persons. The determinants include: social factors, personal factors, economic situations, behavioural factors, aspects of the physical environment, and health and social services. The elements of gender and culture are interwoven through each determinant–their unique impacts to each determinant will be explored. Social exclusion is a prime social determinant of health and the process of social exclusion negatively affects all the determinants (Health Canada, 1996).

Age is not included in Health Canada's determinants of health but it is included here as an important concept. Ageism has been identified in the literature for marginalizing older people and as a key factor to social isolation and exclusion. The older a cohort gets the greater the levels of disability in that group and thus the greater chances of institutionalization as well as possibly the risk of elder abuse due to increased vulnerability (Harbison, 2004).

Income, Income Distribution, and Social Status

Studies show that health status improves at each step up the income and social hierarchy. In addition, societies that are reasonably prosperous and have an equitable distribution of wealth have the healthiest populations, regardless of the amount they spend on health care (Health Canada, 2001). It is thought that higher income and social status generally result in older adults feeling more control and choice in their lives, which are key influences on their health. Many older adults have incomes below the poverty line. Women are more likely than men to fall into this low-income category (Podnieks, 1997). Those older adults who have little economic stability have an increased chance of experiencing poor health and premature death. Poverty increases the risk of social isolation, lack of information, and poor health, particularly for older adults from minority cultures and for older adults with disabilities (MacLeod, 1997). Often older adults living in poverty lack social contacts or community supports, and experience feelings of uselessness, loneliness, dependence, as well as depression (MacLeod, 1997). These challenges can be compounded by histories of abuse, low self-esteem, powerlessness, and health problems caused by abuse. Economic uncertainty due to governmental cutbacks may lead to poverty and the eroding social status and self-esteem of older adults. Studies show that older adults often become deeply depressed and worried about being a burden on society, adding to the feelings of inferiority and loss many older adults feel upon retirement (MacLeod, 1997). Such feelings can trigger a helpless and hopeless attitude, whereby the older person may feel that the abuse they experience is justified and therefore they accept the abusive manner is which they are treated, and do not seek help. Clearly, all of these factors make older persons more vulnerable to abuse, and act as barriers to obtaining appropriate support (Podnieks and Pillemer, 1990).

Social Support Networks

Support and good social relations make an important contribution to health. Social support from families, friends, and communities is associated with better health and equips older adults with the emotional and practical resources they need to cope with growing older. Belonging to social networks makes people feel cared for, loved, esteemed, and valued, providing a powerful protective effect on mental and physical health (Wilkinson and Marmot, 2002). Current social trends have weakened traditional family, friendships, neighborhood and community networks, leaving many families and individuals isolated from natural support systems. Older adults who are isolated socially may have a wide range of health problems and risk factors, which further limit their social support networks, and those of their informal caregivers as well (MacLeod, 1997).

Lack of social support has been linked to abusive behaviour (Anetzberger, 2005). Abused older adults may be more socially isolated and have fewer social contacts than non-abused older adults. Furthermore, when families are isolated from the support of friends and relatives, older members are at a greater risk for abusive behaviour that may be undetected (Podnieks, 1997). The absence of emotional and practical social support varies by social and economic status, and places older adults at an increased risk for abuse and neglect.

Transportation problems in both urban and rural communities can create major barriers to social contact, recreation, and active living for older adults, especially those with disabilities. Lack of transportation is isolating and frustrating for many individuals, which can lead to an increase in health-damaging behaviours such as drug and alcohol dependency, both of which are positively correlated to incidences of abuse. Lack of transportation limits the older adult from accessing appropriate healthcare services, limits participation in social events and religious activity.

Social isolation resulting from loss of significant others, role loss, loss of body image, and cultural/linguistic barriers is linked to poor mental health and to drug and alcohol use (Health Canada, 1994). Identifying social isolation can be a key element in assessing risk for elder abuse and implementing proactive approaches to prevent it. Victims have disclosed that being abused and keeping this a secret intensifies their loneliness and isolation (Podnieks, 1992).

Education and Literacy

Education is an important determinant of health. Health status increases with the level of education. Education increases opportunities for income and job security, equips people with problem-solving skills, and gives people a sense of mastery and control over their lives. Education and literacy also improves one's ability to access and understand information, which are key factors that influence health. Low literacy rates can make it more difficult for older adults to care for their health, and to manage their finances (World Health Organization, 2002). Because these older adults tend to rely on social supports for help with reading and writing, such dependency places them in a precarious situation in which abuse and neglect may evolve. It further inhibits their ability to respond to written care plans or directions.

Education has the potential to be a major factor in risk reduction for abuse but it must be accompanied by other interventions that are applied concurrently to help equalize the power and control balance between older adults and those who interact with them. Training older adults strategies that can be adopted to arm oneself against abuse and access help in abusive situations will enable them to develop "resiliency" to abuse, and must include measures to change those administrative, legal, social, and cultural conditions that foster abuse. Educating children and youth to become aware of the abuse and neglect of older adults places them in a position to prevent it from happening (Podnieks and Baillie, 1995). Increased education will provide all members of society with accurate information about older adults and the aging process itself, helping to overcome the effects of negative myths and will improve overall ageist perceptions, therefore fostering a society in which violence against older adults will not be tolerated.

Employment and Working Conditions

Employment leads to economic stability, which, combined with a healthy work environment, leads to good health. Unemployment, underemployment, and stressful work environments are associated with poor health. Older adults who have control over their working circumstances and fewer stress-related demands of the job are healthier and often live longer than those in more stressful or riskier work activities (Health Canada, 1994). Health is also increased through the effects of workplace supports. Employment and working conditions may impact on the behaviour of the abuser. If the abuser has no control over their work circumstances, and has many stress-related demands on the job, abusive actions may escalate towards the older adult over whom they exert power.

In examining the health determinant of employment and working conditions, it behooves us to consider institutional care and strains and contradictions facing both care providers and their clients. Fonner (1994) asks a critical question: Are the pressures that discourage compassionate care an inevitable product of forces in institutions or are they amenable to change? How can social inclusion be enhanced in such environments?

Currently, in many long-term care facilities, significant proportions of the staff are hired on a casual, floating or part-time basis. These staff may have fewer opportunities to "bond with" residents and get to know them. The use of casual or floating staff can interfere with continuity of care and ability to provide sensitive resident-centred care. Long-term care facilities are challenged to provide care to an increasingly complex resident population–with higher medical, mental health/behavioural, psychosocial, and cognitive needs. Depending on the facility, staff may or may not receive adequate education and training to manage these care challenges appropriately. Inadequate training can lead to use of inappropriate care interventions, contribute to caregiver burnout and increase the risk of abuse (Speer, 2005).

While the complexity of care has increased, so too has the cost to deliver quality care. Yet, long-term care facilities must still operate within tight budgets and rigid policy guidelines. Cost-containment is highly valued and long term care homes are continually challenged to rationalize the best use of resources. However, the very nature of caregiving work, the bulk of which is labour intensive and repetitive, performed by nursing and personal support staff (e.g., Aides, PSWs) means that its value and contribution to organizations and individual health outcomes can be difficult to measure in objective terms. It can be difficult to capture/quantify how many staff members are required to truly meet a resident's physical, psychosocial, behavioural, cognitive, and spiritual needs. As a result, staff ratios may not reflect the true care needs for a resident population. In this environment, the older adult becomes depersonalized, care becomes compartmentalized–a series of tasks to be completed or "done to" the older adult–often not negotiated with the person receiving care (Speer, 2005). This working environment can create stress both for staff and the residents. Time constraints, unit routines and even organizational policies and procedures and legislation can pose considerable barriers to the provision of care that is resident-focused and culturally appropriate. Staff report that the administrative perspective tends to place less value on the interpersonal aspects of care than the functional aspects. Additionally, many frontline staff have limited control in determining organizational activities and exert little control over the structure of their work (Speer, 2005). Caregiving itself, by nature, is highly stressful. Thus, the institutional workplace can be a fertile place for social exclusion and subsequent elder abuse.

Social Environments

Societal values and rules affect the health and well-being of individuals and populations. Social stability, recognition of diversity, good human relationships, and community cohesiveness provide a supportive social environment, which mitigates risks to optimal health. Public policy development and implementation is a social and political process that must consider the diverse and changing needs of older adults, especially women and members of disadvantaged ethnic groups. Social and economic policies and practices must be put into place in order to prevent and appropriately intervene in the abuse and neglect of older adults (Mustard and Frank, 1991).

Inequalities in resource allocation and service delivery are a reality that should not be accepted, as such discrimination only succeeds in the marginalization of the older population. Older adults may not receive health and social services because the services offered are inadequate, unavailable, inaccessible, unknown, or because they do not meet the eligibility criteria, there are language difficulties, and/or lack of transportation. In Canada, there are a disproportionate amount of services available for youth or adults in contrast to the older population. This sends a message to society that as one ages one is not valuable, not worthy of the same health and social protections as other age cohorts. These current political practices breed ageist attitudes that adhere to abuse and neglect as appropriate ways to "deal" with older adults (Podnieks, 2002). A similar example appeared several years ago when a Congressional Hearing concluded that although elder abuse is a very serious problem, widespread in society, spending money on it would "conflict with the needs of children" (U.S. House of Representatives, 1991).

Physical Environments

Physical factors in the natural environment such as air, water, and soil quality are key influences on health. Factors in the human-built environment such as housing, safety, community and road design are also important. It is necessary to prevent injury in the older population because of the increase in the consequences of an injury, which is often more severe and disabling as an individual ages (Ross and Podnieks, 1997). Placing older adults in situations of increased dependency on caregivers can lead to abuse and neglectful situations. Fortunately, most injuries sustained by older adults are preventable. Accidents are the major cause of non-fatal and fatal injuries among Canada's older population and 40 percent of admissions to institutions. They are also the leading cause of fatal injury among older adults (*Toronto Star*, 2001). When the physical environment is made safe and accessible for older adults, both physical and mental health improve, and they remain well and independent (MacLeod, 1997). They are less dependent on others and consequently less susceptible to situations of abuse and neglect.

Safe, accessible and affordable housing is an important aspect of the physical environment. The quality of the environment and housing is important to the health and well-being of older adults because of the increase in the amount of time spent at home. Situations in which older adults are living in close quarters with family members may accelerate abusive and neglectful situations. This is a problem particularly for older adults who are part of low-income families, including many older adults who are immigrants to a country. When older adults are provided with adequate housing or shelter alternatives, when faced with situations of abuse and neglect, it allows them to regain a healthy mental and physical well-being and create a life away from the abuser (Health Canada, 1994).

High proportions of the residents of small towns are older adults because they age in place, while younger cohorts migrate to larger urban centers. This may lead to situations of isolation and a state of dependency on others for assistance because of fewer social services in rural areas. Unfortunately, the loss of independence experienced by some older adults living in rural areas may lead some individuals to take advantage and exploit the older adult. Older adults who live in urban areas experience a different social and physical environment. They may have poorer housing, be more dependent on transportation, have a higher cost of living, and be more susceptible to crime. Fear of crime, especially among those who are economically and socially disadvantaged, can be debilitating, leading to isolation and increased risk of abuse and neglect (MacLeod, 1997).

Personal Health Practices

Personal health practices and coping skills are imperative to maintain health levels. Many studies have shown that older adults who are physically active report a greater sense of subjective well-being, and control over their lives, and are therefore better equipped to cope with life stresses (Health Canada, 1996). An active older adult is capable of defending him/herself from abusive situations both physically and psychologically. They are often more independent, and if threatened, can physically leave the situation of abuse. Having access to fresh nutritious foods plays a key role in this determinant because if an older adult is properly nourished they are more likely to feel well enough to be physically active. Adequate nutrition in older adulthood is essential in maintaining health and preventing or controlling chronic diseases. Nutritional risk factors are associated with the development and progression of many chronic diseases–conversely, good healthy nutrition practices are cited as protective factors in preventing the development of many chronic diseases (such as control of hypertension, obesity, and diabetes) (Worthington-Roberts et al., 1996). Levels of educations and income influence accessibility to safe nutritious foods. In cases of neglect and abuse, the caregiver may be unaware or unable to recognize the needs of the older adult. For example, the older adult may be experiencing difficulty eating due to improper oral care, swallowing difficulties, or lack of and/or poorly fitting dentures, and therefore is unable to consume the nutrition they require. Accessibility to a reliable source of fresh nutritious foods is impacted by many factors including poverty, chemical abuse, and caregiver neglect.

Individual Capacity and Coping Skills

Social environments that enable and support healthy choices and lifestyles, as well as people's knowledge, intentions, behaviours, and coping skills for dealing with life in healthy ways, are key influences on health. It is critical that we consider the impact of various chronic conditions and disabilities that people develop as they age on the person's coping strategy and style, body image, self-perception, and self-efficacy. Coping style will influence the person's attitudes and perceptions of his/her ability to manage the challenges and stressors they encounter. Older adults who develop "hardy" traits and attitudes may experience increased sense of control over their lives, thus protecting them from abusive and neglectful situations. Low self-esteem and stress among older adults reduces their coping skills and places many older adults at risk for abuse and neglect (Podnieks, 1997).

Biology and Genetic Endowment

The genetic endowment of the individual, the functioning of various body systems and the process of development and aging are fundamental determinants of health. Biological differences in sex, and socially constructed gender, influence health on an individual and population basis (Health Canada, 1994). For example, men and women have different life expectancies. The age of onset of the types of disease, illness and conditions, which are prime causes of morbidity, disability and mortality, are different for men and women. The growth of the elderly population is characterized by gender differences. The proportion of women grew steadily and rapidly during the postwar period, while the proportion of men, particularly those over 80 years of age, declined. The preponderance of older women with healthcare problems; their concentration in institutional settings, the roles of their daughters and daughter-in-laws as caregivers; and, the continuing level of poverty among elderly women are all issues relating to abuse and neglect. Similarly, persons with disabilities who live in their own home or in institutions and who rely on others for assistance with their care are vulnerable to abuse (Health Canada, 1996).

Health Services

Health services, particularly those designed to maintain and promote health and prevent disease, contribute to health. Services that educate people about health risks and healthy choices support healthy living. Those that encourage and assist in the adoption of healthy living practices and support independent living also make a contribution to health. Community environmental health services that help to ensure the safety of food, water and living environments and health care services designed to treat illness and restore health or functioning also contribute to keeping people healthy (Health Canada, 1996). The aging population is growing at a rate unprecedented in history and will continue to do so into the next century. The population over the age of 85 will increase most dramatically, many of whom will be disabled. In addition, other persons with disabilities require specialized services conducive to health and well-being. The current economic and health climate includes a commitment to wellness programs and community services. This commitment, however, is counterbalanced by downsizing and fiscal restraint. New definitions of essential and non-essential services are emerging. More is expected for less. Central to all discussions regarding health services should be recognition of the entitlement of elderly and/or disabled persons to health services (Dow Pittaway, 1998). Older adults who do have health services available to them may be identified as victims or potential victims of elder mistreatment. Intervention can then be implemented and ultimately contribute to the safety and security of older persons.

Gender and Culture

It is acknowledged that culture and gender have a cross-cutting, influential effect on all the other health determinants. Gender refers to the many different roles, personality traits, attitudes, behaviours, relative powers and influences which society assigns to the two sexes (Health Canada, 2001). Culture comes from both the personal history and wider situational, social, political, geographic, and economic factors. Gender can have a profound effect on such factors as social status, how older people access healthcare, meaningful work, and leisure/recreational opportunities and other resources. Gender and cultural characteristics affect how older adults maintain their personal and group identity, status, and traditions, all of which contribute to the health of the individual and population. While many studies have found that older women are most likely to be victims of abuse, gender influences may also differ according to the type of abuse (Podnieks, 1997). In Canada, for example, material abuse is equally common among males and females living alone, and although males are more likely to be physically abused, physical abuse by males toward females tends to be more violent (Podnieks, 1990). Vulnerability can make it more difficult for either a man or woman to escape or report abuse. However, it is ageist social attitudes towards older adults that are probably greater factors in the under-detection and under-reporting of abuse. Ageist attitudes reinforce and perpetuate an increased vulnerability to abuse and neglect in older adults (Podnieks, 1997).

The underlying premise of gender as a key determinant of health assumes that older women are more vulnerable to gender-based physical violence and gender bias (Dow Pittaway, 1998). This premise was substantiated in the Dow Pittaway survey (1998), which found a higher proportion of women (79.2%) compared to men (20.8%) were physically abused. Aronson, Thornwell, and Willows (1995) and Neysmith (1995) feel the term abuse masks the link between abuse against women and the relative powerlessness of women throughout their lives: studies of elder abuse must link current abuse to structured social inequalities. HelpAge International (2001) poignantly describes how women are being excluded from dialogue and planning to improve their well-being and environment. Thus, older women are discriminated against and do not receive their fair share of resources.

Culture is considered a key determinant to health, assuming that some persons or groups may face additional health risks due to their socio-economic circumstances, which are influenced by dominant cultural values. The social environment, which is determined in large measure by mainstream culture, may perpetuate conditions such as marginalization, stigmatization, loss or devaluation of language, and lack of access to culturally appropriate healthcare and services, all resulting in social exclusion (Dow Pittaway, 1998; Podnieks, 1997). There is little question that those factors can severely impact the degree of social isolation and subsequent mistreatment experienced by older people. Negative societal attitudes and ignorance of the aging process may result in a climate that is favorable to abusive situations. Through an understanding of individual cultures in society we can work toward an understanding of the barriers that may prevent and discourage older adults and their families from seeking help or disclosing information to service providers.

THE INCLUSION LENS

Having examined the determinants of health and how they can provide a framework within which to situate elder abuse, an intervention strategy is now presented.

The Inclusion Lens[1] provides government, non-government organizations (NGOs), community groups, and social agencies a way of doing something to promote social and economic inclusion, and in doing so contributes to the prevention of elder abuse. In using the Inclusion Lens, professionals and practitioners can analyze the source of exclusion of a population or a community concern, identify some solutions leading toward inclusion and develop a plan of action.

What Are Social and Economic Inclusion?

Inclusion is a term that is familiar to most people in their everyday lives. We feel included or excluded, from family, neighborhood, or community activities. Inclusion and exclusion have also been recognized as social issues in Europe since the 1970s, where they have become central features of public policies. Social and economic exclusion and inclusion have recently become the focus of attention among those who are concerned about poverty and its many negative effects on people.

What Is an Inclusion Lens?

A lens is an aid to improve vision. It can also provide a new way to look at root causes of old problems, like poverty, discrimination, abuse, disadvantage, and disability. The term "Inclusion Lens" is a shorthand way of looking at social and economic exclusion and inclusion. The Inclusion Lens is a tool for analyzing legislation, policies, programs, and practices to determine whether they promote the social and economic inclusion of individuals, families, and community. It will open up minds to new ways of thinking, and open doors to new solutions for old problems. Ultimately, it provides a new way to encourage change that will transform society.

The Inclusion Lens is designed for use by policy makers, program managers, and community leaders who work in the context of social and economic exclusion, in both public and non-profit sectors. It could also be a tool for activists in social movements, such as women and people with disabilities, and community developers working toward healthy, sustainable communities. It provides a method for analyzing both the conditions of family and solutions that promote inclusion. It also provides a way of beginning to plan for inclusion (Shookner, 2002).

Why Is a Tool Needed?

Social and economic exclusion and inclusion have emerged as new ways of understanding poverty and disadvantage, and their impact on health and well-being, by creating a shared understanding across sectors and jurisdictions as the basis for action. One of the overarching objectives is to influence the development of healthy public policies and programs which address the determinants of health, and which promote social and economic inclusion. Strategies to promote social and economic inclusion call for actions that respond to the individual, family, community, and societal concerns. Complex problems require complex solutions. Action is required from many sectors in society in addressing the systemic nature of exclusion. Policy makers need tools and methods to create public policies that are inclusive. These tools help them translate the concepts of social and economic exclusion and inclusion into concrete terms that can then be fed into the public policy development process.

The Inclusion Lens provides a way to begin the dialogue with excluded groups such as seniors, raise awareness about how exclusion works, and identify steps to move towards policies, programs and practices that will be inclusive (Shookner, 2002). The challenge for readers of this article is to advocate for mistreated older persons by addressing elder abuse through a social inclusion model: How can we reframe our present approaches to become more creative in addressing and managing elder abuse cases through the Inclusion Lens? The following description of the tool illuminates the way for health and human service providers to become involved in the process.

How Can the Inclusion Lens Be Used?

This new tool may be used in a variety of settings to analyze conditions that exclude people, communities and populations from participating in the social and economic benefits of society. Governments at all levels can use the Inclusion Lens to analyze legislation, policies, and programs to determine whether these exclude or include people who are marginalized, disadvantaged, impoverished, or discriminated against. Non-Government organizations can use the Inclusion Lens to find out if the policies, programs, and practices they use exclude or include people in vulnerable situations. Community groups can use the Inclusion Lens for planning, development, and social action to address the sources of exclusion in communities and public policies, and pointing toward solutions that will be inclusive.

Dimensions of Exclusion and Inclusion

Social and economic exclusion and inclusion can be seen along several dimensions–*cultural, economic, functional, participatory, physical, political, structural*, and *relational*. There are many elements to exclusion and inclusion that should be considered in analyzing a policy, program, or practice. The key questions listed below are not intended to comprise a complete list, but to stimulate readers to think about which of these may apply to their particular situations. Some elements may relate to more than one dimension. Additional elements may also be identified.

Values: The Foundation for Inclusion

The Inclusion Lens needs a foundation of values to guide how it is used. These values arise from the work that has taken place in Atlantic Canada on social and economic exclusion and inclusion:

- Social Justice–Distribution of the social and economic resources of society for the benefit of all people.
- Valuing Diversity–Recognition and respect for the diversity of cultures, races, ethnicity, languages, abilities, age, and sexual orientation; valuing all contributions of both men and women to the social, economic, and cultural vitality of society
- Opportunities for Choice–Respect for the right of individuals to make choices that affect their lives
- Entitlement to Rights and Services–Recognition of universal entitlement to rights and services as set out in the human rights covenants, charters, and legislation.
- Working Together–Building common interests and relationships as the basis for actions to achieve shared goals.

Creating Your Own Lens–Think about creating your own inclusion lens. Answer the following questions about exclusion and inclusion using a participatory process that involves people who are excluded. Fill in your own template (not included) with the elements of exclusion and inclusion appropriate to your situation.

Key Questions: This view of social and economic exclusion and inclusion suggests key questions that could be asked about any policy, program, or practice.

Questions about Exclusion: Who is being excluded? From what? How do you see exclusion working? Who benefits from exclusion?

Questions about Inclusion: Who are the people to be included? How do you see inclusion working? Who benefits from inclusion?

Questions About Social and Economic Exclusion:

1. Who is being excluded? From what?
2. What are the sources of exclusion in the policy, program, or practice?
3. What impacts do the current programs or policies have on promoting exclusion?
4. What is the impact of exclusion on people in the short term?
5. Are there long-term impacts?
6. What are the costs of exclusion? Who bears them?
7. Who benefits from exclusion?
8. Who has the responsibility, jurisdiction to address the sources of exclusion?
9. Who are the people to be included?
10. What legislations, policies, programs, or practices would promote inclusion?
11. What impacts do the current programs or policies have on promoting inclusion?
12. What are the measures of inclusion?
13. Who benefits from inclusion?
14. Who needs to be involved in the solutions?
15. What processes are needed to make the solutions work?
16. What are the desired outcomes of inclusion in the short term, medium term, long term?

Looking Through the Inclusion Lens

Questions to Ask:

1. How will the policy or program increase or decrease discrimination on the basis of gender, race, age, culture, or ethnicity?
2. How will the policy or program increase or decrease personal income and resources available for people to participate in social and economic activity and promote income equity?
3. How will the policy or program increase or decrease isolation and access to resources?
4. How will the policy or program increase or decrease opportunities for participation in decision-making?
5. How will the policy or program add or remove barriers to common spaces, safe environments, and social interaction?
6. How will the policy or program protect or compromise the rights of people?
7. How will the policy or program increase or decrease opportunities for personal development and social support?
8. How will the policy or program increase or reduce access to resources and programs for excluded groups?

Developing Your Action Plan

By now readers are equipped with an analysis of social and economic exclusion for a selected population, policy, or program and pointers toward solutions that promote inclusion. The next step is to develop an action plan.

Key Considerations:

1. Population.
2. Policy or program.
3. Key strategies.
4. Who is responsible?
5. Roles of partners or collaborators. Who takes the lead?
6. Processes of participation.
7. Resources needed. From where/whom?
8. Timelines.
9. Measures of progress.
10. Desired outcomes.

Taking Action for Inclusion

By using this Inclusion Lens, readers have analyzed the sources of exclusion of a population or community of concern, identified solutions leading toward inclusion, and developed a plan to get started. Congratulations!

Anyone can take action toward a more inclusive society–socially and economically. People in government, non-government organizations, community groups, and social agencies can do something to promote social and economic inclusion. This tool will help you to work toward your goals.

For more information about the Inclusion Lens, please contact Malcolm Shookner, Population Health Research Centre, Dalhousie University, Halifax Nova Scotia. E-mail: Malcolm.Shookner@dal.ca, phone: (902) 494-1590, fax: (902) 494-3594.

More information about social and economic inclusion can be obtained on the following websites: www.pph-atlantic.ca–Population and Public Health Branch, Atlantic Regional Office, Health Canada or www.medicine. dal.ca/acewh–Atlantic Centre for Excellence for Women's Health.

INCLUSION LENS AND THE DETERMINANTS OF HEALTH: POWERFUL TOOLS TO FOCUS UNDERSTANDING OF, AND APPROACHES TO ELDER ABUSE

The idea of 'social inclusion' is now the central legitimating concept of social policy in Europe and elsewhere. There is a general agreement that inclusion is a good thing, and that exclusion is a bad thing, both because it is unfair, and because it damages social cohesion. Social inclusion and exclusion have been variously defined. One example of inclusion is provided by Health Canada (2000), which defines it as ". . . the capacity and willingness of our society to keep all groups within reach of what we expect as a society–the social commitment and investments necessary to ensure that socially and economically vulnerable people are within reach of our common aspirations, common life and its common wealth." de Haan (1999) offers the following definition, "Exclusion is primarily defined as the rupture of the social bond–which is cultural and moral–between the individual and society. National solidarity implies political right and duty."

Social and economic inclusion provides a framework that includes all of the determinants of health. International evidence has established that economic inequality is a powerful determinant of health. The wider the gap between the rich and the poor, the poorer the health status of the entire population. Adequate income, education, and a network of relationships enable people to participate as valued members of society (Guildford, 2000).

The experience of exclusion can be seen through the interplay of the determinants of health: "Each linkage deepens the experience of exclusion, and over the entire life cycle, the depth of exclusion is reinforced . . . The linking of low access to resources, low social status, low levels of education, and healthy child development, high levels of racial intolerance and unemployment, fragmented social networks, and limited access to health services, deepens the exclusion" (Guildford, 2000). Gilbert (2003) reminds us that social inclusion is a complex and challenging concept that cannot be reduced to a single dimension or meaning. As advocates for older persons, we must call for the strongest possible statement condemning violence against older people, as an infringement of their most basic human rights. The extent and nature of violence perpetrated against older men and women is only just becoming apparent. The issue is now being talked about to a greater extent because older people have the courage to speak out. Older people are telling us that they view old age with anxiety and fear, not only because of increasing poverty, but the potential increasing dependency on others and consequent vulnerability to physical, sexual, and psychological abuse.

In applying the determinants of health framework to social inclusion in addressing elder abuse, we need to integrate our knowledge with that of the Determinants of Active Aging, a renewed perspective on population aging initiated by the World Health Organization (WHO, 2001). These include: independence, participation, care, self-fulfillment, care, and dignity. Decisions are based on an understanding of how these determinants of active aging influence the way that individuals and populations age. Policy action to address these determinants is required in three areas: health and independence, productivity, and protection (WHO, 2001).

The merits of the Inclusion Lens as a tool for elder abuse prevention and intervention have been discussed at several recent educational and scientific conferences, and have received preliminary support from researchers and human service professionals alike. For example, one conference participant felt the inclusion lens would provide a unique opportunity for case managers to work through elder abuse cases, ensure values are not being overlooked, provide a chance to expand vision/focus on elder abuse and help to shape agency/organizational goals.

CONCLUSION

A focus on the determinants of health provide us with an opportunity to conduct research that may facilitate intervention in both individual and family practice and should ultimately influence policy. Much of the elder abuse literature has centred upon the victim or abuser or both (Hudson and Johnson, 1986). Many explanations and interventions are predominantly designed for micro or individual levels. While this micro approach is essential in practice we need to expand our framework for analyzing elder abuse to a more macro perspective–to a structural perspective–so that we do not run the risk of regarding elder abuse as a private, rather than public concern. Silver (1999) describes a whole range of approaches to monitoring social exclusion from macro to micro levels. In order to understand elder abuse as a social problem, it is essential to review how the determinants of health influence abuse and social responses to abuse. Clearly, the social inclusion lens shows that older people from diverse backgrounds need to be involved in partnerships in research, practice and decision-making levels, in order to increase the cultural sensitivity that is needed to reduce and eliminate marginalization of older people. Individuals who may be disadvantaged due to their age, gender, education, social support network, health status, and culture need to be included in organizational structures and in the development and delivery of services, if society is ever to be sensitive to the needs of all its members (Dow Pittaway, 1998). The focus on the determinants of health can enhance health promotion and lead to social inclusion. It is hoped that analysis of these health determinants–as they relate specifically to elder abuse–will promote more critical reflection on elder abuse as a social problem at the macro level.

Social inclusion may be viewed as a social lens through which to understand social well-being, equality, and citizenship (Gilbert, 2003). Elder abuse is a complex, disturbing problem, which goes to the very core of human rights and freedoms. What constitutes violence, abuse, and neglect are still ill defined–we know that violence is the quintessential threat to individual safety and social stability, but there is little clarity about how we can understand and deal with violence itself (Health and Human Rights, 2003). The mapping of various dimensions of social exclusion/inclusion is helpful and important (de Haan, 1999). This paper attempts to contribute to the knowledge base on elder abuse. It is hoped that it might inspire and facilitate the increased cooperation, innovation and commitment of those working in the field. All efforts need to be directed towards the elimination of all forms of abuse, neglect and discrimination of older persons.

NOTES

1. *The Inclusion Lens: Workbook for Looking at Social and Economic Exclusion and Inclusion.* (2002). Produced by Malcolm Shookner, Population Health Research Centre, Dalhousie University, for the Population and Public Health Branch, Atlantic Regional Office, Health Canada. Reprinted with Permission. Please send comments to

Malcolm Shookner at *Malcolm.shookner@dal.ca.* or by phone: (902) 494-1590 or fax: (902) 494-3594.

REFERENCES

Anetzberger, J. (2005). (Ed.), *The Clinical Management of Elder Abuse.* The Haworth Press, Inc., Binghamton, NY.

Aronson, J., Thornwell, C., and Williams, K. (1995). Wife assault in old age: Coming out of obscurity. *Canadian Journal on Aging,* 14 (Suppl.), 73-88.

Atlantic Centre for Excellence in Women's Health, *Inclusion Project Information Kit,* Halifax, 2000.

Blair, Tony, Prime Minister Speech, December 8, 1997.

Brownell, P. (2003). The Madrid 2002 Plan of Action: Global Aging and 9/11. *Journal of International Social Welfare Policy.* XIX, 1:15-25.

de Haan, A. (1999). *Social Exclusion: Towards a Holistic Understanding of Deprivation.* Paper presented to Villa Borsig Workshop Series 1999: Inclusion, Justice, and Poverty Reduction, Deutsche Stiftung für Internationale Entwicklung 1999.

de Haan, A. (1998). Social exclusion: An alternative concept for the study of deprivation? *IDS Bulletin,* 20:1.

Dow Pittaway, E. (1998). *Collaboration and Inclusion Leading to a Prevalence Study of Abuse.* Paper presented at Linking Ontario to the Broader Elder Abuse Community. Toronto, Canada. March 3, 1998.

Fonner, N. (1994). *The Caregiving Dilemma.* University of California Press, Berkely, CA.

Gilbert, N. (2003). *Laidlaw Foundation's Perspective on Social Inclusion: What Do We Know and Where Do We Go? Building a Social Research Inclusion Agenda.* CCSD Conference. March 28, 2003. Toronto, Canada.

Guildford, J. (2000). *Making the Case for Social and Economic Inclusion.* Population and Public Health Branch, Atlantic Regional Office, Health Canada: Halifax.

Harbison, J. (2004). Dalhousie University, Maritime School of Social Work, unpublished document.

Health Canada (1994). *Population Health Approach: Key Determinants of Health.* Ottawa Charter for Health Promotion.

Health Canada (1996). *A Discussion Paper Towards a Common Understanding.* July 1996.

Health Canada (2000). *Key Learning Two from PPHB Atlantic's Work on Social and Economic Inclusion 1998-2000,* Population and Public Health Branch, Atlantic Regional Office, Health Canada, Halifax 2000.

Health Canada (2001). *The Population Health Template: Key Elements and Actions That Define a Population Health Approach,* Population and Public Health Branch, Strategic Policy Secretariat, Health Canada, Ottawa, July 2001.

Health and Human Rights: An International Journal (2003). *Special Focus: Violence, Health, and Human Rights.* Vol. 6, no. 2.

HelpAge International (2000). *The Mark of a Noble Society.* Human Rights and Older People. London, UK.

HelpAge International (2001). *Equal Treatment, Equal Rights.* Ten Actions to End Age Discrimination. London, UK.

Hudson, M., and Johnson, T. (1986). Elder Abuse and Neglect: A Review of the Literature. *The Annual Review of Gerontology and Geriatrics*, 6, 81-134.

MacLeod, L. (1997). *Toward Healthy-Aging Communities: A Population Health Approach*. Prepared for Division of Aging and Seniors, Population Health Directorate, Health Promotion Branch, Health Canada.

Maritime Centre for Excellence for Women's Health (2001). Dalhousie University. Basic Information about Social and Economic Inclusion.

Maslow, A. (1970). *Toward a Psychology of Being* (2nd Edition). New York: Harper & Row.

McPerson, B.D. (1998). *Aging as a Social Process–An Introduction to Individual and Population Aging: Third Edition*. Harcourt Brace & Company, Canada.

Mustard, F. J., and Frank, J. (1991). The Determinants of Health. *Canadian Institute for Advanced Research Publication #5*, Toronto, Canada.

Neysmith, S. (1995). Power in Relationships of Trust: A Feminist Analysis of Elder Abuse. In McLean, M. (Ed.), *Abuse and Neglect of Older Canadians: Strategies for Change*. Toronto: Thompson Educational Publishing, 1995.

Neysmith, S., and Edwardh, J. (1984). Economic dependency in the 1980s: Its impact on third world's elderly. *Ageing and Society*. 4:1.

Podnieks, E. (2002). *Determinants of Active Aging*. Paper presented at the Second World Assembly on Ageing. Madrid, Spain. April 2002.

Podnieks, E. (1997). *Relationship of Health Determinants of Abuse and Neglect of Older Canadians*. Presented at the 16th World Congress on Gerontology, Adelaide, Australia.

Podnieks, E., and Baillie, F. (1995). Education as the Key to Prevention of Elder Abuse and Neglect. In McLean, M. (Ed.), *Abuse and Neglect of Older Canadians: Strategies for Change*. Toronto: Thompson Educational Publishing, 1995.

Podnieks, E. (1992). Emerging Themes from a follow-up study of Canadian victims of elder abuse. *Journal of Elder Abuse & Neglect*, 4 (1)2, 59-111.

Podnieks, E., and Pillemer, K. (1990). *National Survey on Abuse of the Elderly in Canada*. Ryerson University, Toronto, Ontario, Canada.

Ross, M., and Podnieks, E. (1997). *The Determinants of Health: A Synergy Process of Learning*. Paper presented at the Conference: Adults with Vulnerability: Addressing Abuse and Neglect. January 1997. Toronto, Canada.

Shookner, M. (2002). *An Inclusion Lens: Workbook for Looking at Social and Economic Exclusion and Inclusion*. Population Health Research Centre, Dalhousie University, for the Population and Public Health Branch, Atlantic Regional Office, Health Canada, Halifax, NS.

Silver, H. (1999). *Social Exclusion and Social Solidarity: Three Paradigms*. IILS Discussion Papers no. 69. ILO, Geneva.

Speer, S. (2005). Interview notes, February 2005, Toronto, Canada.

Toronto Star (2001). Fall Safe. December 28, 2001.

U.S. House of Representatives, Select Committee on Aging (1991). *Elder Abuse: What Can Be Done?* Washington, DC: US Congress.

Wilkinson, R., and Marmot, M. (2002). *Social Determinants of Health: The Solid Facts*. Health Canada: Healthy Cities.

World Health Organization (2001). *Health and Aging: A Discussion Paper.* Department of Health Promotion, Non-Communicable Disease Prevention and Surveillance. Geneva, Switzerland.

Worthington-Roberts, B.S., and Williams, S.R. (1996). *Nutrition Throughout the Life Cycle: Third Edition.* WCB McGraw-Hill, USA.

PRACTICE

Self-Determination and Elder Abuse:
Do We Know Enough?

L. René Bergeron, MSW, PhD

SUMMARY. This article explores the principle of self-determination as it relates to victims of elder abuse and neglect. Using newspaper accounts and cases from the author's practice and consulting files, various factors influencing the professional's interpretation of this principle are explored. The notion that self-determination allows victims of abuse and neglect to refuse intervention is challenged. The author concludes that the principle of self-determination and the notion of competency are overly simplified in the social work and elder abuse literature and may be misused by allowing abused older victims to choose to remain in often life-threatening situations. Special focus is given to Adult Protection Service worker, but the author asserts that protecting older people, assisting in creative interventions and developing needed services is a shared professional responsibility. *[Article copies available for a fee from The Haworth Document Delivery Service: 1-800-HAWORTH. E-mail address: <docdelivery@haworthpress.com> Website: <http://www.HaworthPress.com> © 2006 by The Haworth Press, Inc. All rights reserved.]*

[Haworth co-indexing entry note]: "Self-Determination and Elder Abuse: Do We Know Enough?" Bergeron, L. René. Co-published simultaneously in *Journal of Gerontological Social Work* (The Haworth Press, Inc.) Vol. 46, No. 3/4, 2006, pp. 81-102; and: *Elder Abuse and Mistreatment: Policy, Practice, and Research* (ed: M. Joanna Mellor, and Patricia Brownell) The Haworth Press, Inc., 2006, pp. 81-102. Single or multiple copies of this article are available for a fee from The Haworth Document Delivery Service [1-800-HAWORTH, 9:00 a.m. - 5:00 p.m. (EST). E-mail address: docdelivery@haworthpress.com].

KEYWORDS. Elder abuse, elder neglect, self-determination, decision-making, duty-to-protect, competency, adult protection, ethical responsibility

Newspaper Headline: "Judge, lawyer fight elderly neglect. Cases show agency did little to fix elderly's deplorable condition." *The Dallas Morning News*, June 13, 2004.

Adult Protective Service Worker: "The client has the right to make bad decisions." (Bergeron, 1998)

Working with elders suffering from abuse is an important area of interest for the profession of social work. Abused older people are a disenfranchised segment of society needing advocacy to both ensure their protection from continued abuse and their right to self-determine. Nationally, the primary function of taking reports of suspected elder abuse, investigating the reports, and providing intervention when reports are substantiated belongs to Adult Protection Service (APS) agencies. APS practice subscribes to the values and ethics of social work (Simon, 1992; Mixson, 1995) and APS agencies, although they use a staff of mixed degrees, hire many trained social workers. Social workers are encouraged by the National Association of Social Workers to consider entering practice settings that service older clients and are committed to the enhancement of the health and welfare of the growing population of older Americans. However, both the APS protection field and the profession of social work continue to grapple with the notion of client self-determination when servicing competent older adults in compromising situations who refuse interventions to reduce or alleviate abuse or neglect.

Mental incompetence of elder victims is typically cited as the only reason APS workers should disregard an elder's right-to-choose, even if that choice maintains the elder in an unsafe situation. However, the notion of competency and the principle of self-determination are often simplified in the elder abuse literature, and elder protection laws do not provide clear directives regarding terms of competency and self-determination. This lack of directives allows for variances in APS practice interventions and justifies APS workers' closing cases when abused or neglected clients "refuse" services. Victims' right-to-refuse intervention if they are deemed competent appears to override APS workers' duty-to-protect. Yet, APS agencies are held accountable for the outcome of such cases regardless of the victim's competency status.

Protecting elders is not only the responsibility of APS agencies, but is also an ethical responsibility of all professionals who interface with elderly clients.

Mandated reporters of elder abuse and neglect are typically cited in protection laws as being "social workers, physicians, nurses, and law enforcement or police officers, mental health professionals, nursing home personnel, dentists, and more rarely, personnel of financial institutions" (St. James, 2001, 133). Yet, many mandated reporters do not report their suspicions of elder abuse for several reasons (Bergeron, 2003; St. James, 2001). They may be unaware of the reporting law of their state or they may be fearful of losing client/patient rapport if it becomes known it was they who filed the report. They may fail to screen for abuse or fail to recognize abuse when confronted by it. Their perception of elderly people may give them a higher tolerance of abuse (e.g., the notion of ageism). And they may hold the belief that the elder has the right to live however he or she chooses regardless of the severity of the abusive situation (Bergeron, 2004).

Protecting elders, assisting in creative interventions, and developing needed services is a professional community responsibility. Therefore, the understanding all professionals have of the elder's right to self-determination when in abusive or neglectful situations is very important to the well-being of older people, their families, and the community in which they live. It is, however, absolutely critical for the APS workers charged in responding to suspected abuse reports to have a clear sense of the meaning of self-determination in conjunction with their duty-to-protect.

Understanding how self-determination interfaces with other practice values is found in the NASW Code of Ethics (NASW, 2000). This Code provides standards and global values and principles to assist and guide social work practitioners in complex client situations (NASW, 2000). The Code emphasizes that social workers demonstrate respecting the dignity and worth of people by valuing the individual's right to self-determine, empowering the client's own change capacity, and responding to a duty to the broader society when resolving client interests (NASW, 2000). Additionally, the Code balances the principle of self-determination if, in the social worker's assessment, the client is at risk to him or herself or to others (1.02). The Code also addresses impaired client decision-making, stating that social workers need to preserve the rights and interests of clients who cannot make informed decisions (1.14). Several guidelines for the termination of services are cited in the Code as well, stating that client abandonment should be avoided and all factors of the case carefully considered before terminating (1.16). The need to move beyond one's own professional expertise is also addressed in the Code. Social workers, it is stated, should seek interdisciplinary collaboration when it will contribute to those decisions affecting the well-being of clients (2.03), and should use consultation when it is in the best interest of the client (2.05). Social workers should make referrals to other professionals when outside expertise is necessary for case resolution or to assist in the case progress (2.06). Thus, these guidelines suggest that self-determination is not the only guiding principle professionals should reference in practice when working with competent elders suffering from abuse and neglect who refuse services. Unfortunately, the Code does not tell social workers *how* to incorporate these guidelines when faced with difficult client situations, except that each case must be decided by the social worker through critical and ethical decision-making (NASW, 2000). The strong link of APS practice to the field of social work suggests that this Code may be useful in helping APS workers to understand the role of self-determination in elder protection. Likewise, examining how APS workers interpret the principle of self-determination and their duty-to-protect may greatly enhance the overall social work profession's understanding of this very important, complex and ethical standard.

In this article I explore the principle of self-determination for social workers involved with elderly clients experiencing abuse, exploitation, or neglect with a special focus on APS workers charged with responding to such allegations. I outline factors needing consideration and ask those who practice in the elder abuse protection field and those of us who research elder abuse this question about self-determination: "Do we know enough?"

OVERVIEW

Every state has either voluntary or involuntary reporting laws to protect elders from abuse, neglect, and exploitation. Reports of suspected cases of elder abuse are responded to by a designated state agency. Many states refer to the elder protection agency as Adult Protective Services (APS) because protection laws include two groups: people 18 years of age and older with disabilities and people who are elderly, typically defined as age 60 and older. This article only addresses the aged population. The National Adult Protective Services Association (NAPSA) has developed Ethical Principles (NAPSA, 2004) with client self-determination as the guiding value. These Principles are reflective of the APS laws, which ensure client autonomy and the right of every client to self-determine. Additionally, the Principles cite the rights of adults to be safe and retain their civil and constitutional rights. Most APS laws require that an elderly person must be "vulnerable" in some way to mandate an investigation and, if competent, that he or she retains the right to refuse services, even if abuse has been substantiated. In this way states try to respect individuals' right to privacy and their right to live without state interference. The Principles and APS laws are an attempt to prevent APS workers from making decisions about abused clients that are "convenient" in resolving the threat, or to limit the power to "override" victims' desires. Thus, APS workers find themselves confronted with working in a system that charges them to protect older citizens while simultaneously upholding victims' right-to-choose.

However, abused clients' decisions to accept or refuse interventions should not be based solely on what the client wants in that moment in time with the professional. Instead, professionals, in particular APS workers, must have a comprehensive knowledge of the client's life history, a deep understanding of client competency, a holistic definition of self-determination, as well as knowledge of the laws in the civil and criminal courts designed to protect people of every age. They must also have the ability to practice using the Code of Ethics and to think critically about these complex values and principles that govern their working with people. Without this understanding and the ability to translate it into practice, professionals may make inappropriate decisions to withhold reporting a suspected case to protective services, or be uncommitted in including the population of abused elders in their repertoire of public services, or leave clients in life-threatening situations after substantiating that abuse or neglect exist. Such decisions may result in severe harm or death to the client, present a liability to the agency, and certainly expose those cases having dire consequences to public scrutiny via the media, oftentimes creating public misunderstanding. This type of media coverage may also fuel a distrust of the profession of social work and of the APS system as a viable means to resolve elder abuse and neglect as suggested in the newspaper heading at the beginning of this article. Furthermore, if the public and other key professionals in protection work, such as law enforcement and judges, lose faith in the expertise of APS agencies to resolve abusive situations, APS agencies may lose part or all of this important societal function. And I would suggest that should that occur, older clients would be greatly restricted in their ability to self-determine. The dilemma then in elder protection work is the understanding professionals have of the principle of self-determination to judge how much intervention preserves individual choice while providing victim protection.

TYPES OF ABUSE

Elder abuse presents itself in several forms and often in a combination of forms. An elder may be physically abused, meaning a perpetrator intentionally inflicts injury or pain on a victim. Emotional abuse of an elder refers to a perpetrator's use of intimidation to produce fear, humiliation, or helplessness in an elder. An elder may be sexually abused by a perpetrator who has forced unwanted, or undesired sexual encounters, including showing the elder sexually explicit pictures, videos or having the elder observing live sexual acts. Neglect refers to the unmet basic living and medical needs of the elder and may also include abandoning an elderly person not capable of providing self-care. Neglect of an elder may be self-neglectful (no perpetrator involved) or may be a result of a caretaker withholding needed care. Self-neglect also includes the collection of either valuable or worthless items, or the collection of animals without the provision to provide them with proper care. This "collecting" of stuff or animals is referred to as hoarding (Thomas, 1997) and results in health and safety issues for the client and, in some cases, for the immediate community. Financial exploitation refers to a perpetrator's illegal use or the misuse of an elder's income, or any form of assets, including one's home, for self-gain.

MITIGATING FACTORS OF SELF-DETERMINATION

Self-determination is viewed as an individual's right to make decisions affecting his or her life; it is a principle that promotes self-realization (Ewalt and Mokuau, 1995). However, Callahan (1997) examined self-determination within the framework of assisted suicide. He makes a very strong argument that policies or laws permitting individuals the right to participate in assisted suicide do not consider the interrelationships of ". . . the rights of the individual and those of the 'common good' or the well-being of society at large" (243). He explains that social work's subscription to self-determination as the premier principle of practice is an "American" notion based on the high value of individualism in this country and that it lacks an integration of community needs. He also ascertains that this assertion of individual rights removes social workers from fully examining clients in the context of their environment, necessary if one is to practice from an ecological perspective.

Ewalt and Mokuau (1995) support Callahan's notion that as a profession we have interpreted self-determination to imply individual choice over community good. They uphold that this is a middle-class view of white Americans and often does not serve the best interest of people-of-color or other cultural groups that value group well-being above individual desires or self-gain.

Callahan suggests that this minimization of the community as a value and the investment in individualism as the premier value is contributing to the dramatic rise of depression among people (1997). His suggestion is important because depression isolates people from fully participating in society and in making appropriate choices.

Ganzini, Lee, Heintz, and Bloom speak about the difficulty of servicing elderly patients who are depressed:

A patient who feels worthless may refuse treatment out of a desire to cease to be a burden. A hopeless patient may believe that a bad outcome [from the proposed intervention], although statistically unlikely, is certain to occur in her case. A patient with poor motivation may believe that he is unable to mount the energy to participate in painful or invasive therapies . . . Feelings of guilt, personal inadequacy, and hopelessness may cause the patient to be unconvinced of the possibility of present or future recovery. (1993, p. 47)

With this in mind, consider the hoarding case reported in *The Arizona Daily Star* (Burchell & Swedlund, 2004). Fannie Claussen, 86-years-old, lives alone, and within a small area of her front yard, sleeping in a lawn chair. This is because her mobile home was boarded up and padlocked by city officials due to health and safety issues. The newspaper reported that she is in a crime-ridden neighborhood and is exposed to 100-degree heat. She has no doctor, although she supposedly moved to Arizona because of an asthmatic condition. She lives like this because of hoarding behaviors–both her yard and her mobile home are filled with "stuff," including 15 cats, two box turtles, and two desert tortoises. Ranges of services have been offered to clean up both her yard and home to make it livable, but she refuses. The only services listed as accepted by her are meals-on-wheels and a one-night stay in a hotel. The APS agency investigating this case asserts that it is her right to refuse services and live like this because she is competent. Neighbors express concern and outrage that nothing is being done. Ms. Claussen states she could clean up the mess herself if people would leave her alone (Burchell & Swedlund, 2004). Does this woman have the right to live like this where others in the community can see her condition and watch her demise–a kind of ultimate "reality show"? Must neighbors tolerate the deterioration of her home and yard and perhaps have their yards become homes to feral cats? Should neighbors have to witness a violent crime because of her vulnerability? What, if any, is *her* obligation to the community? Is her behavior contributing to the demise of the neighborhood, or the devaluation of surrounding property? Further, does her decision to live like this reflect a competent choice? Or is part of her refusal of services based on some level of depression or hopelessness? Is there a level of intervention that can improve her life, protect neighbors from witnessing an overtly neglectful situation without a total disregard of her wishes? End-of-life literature addresses some of these questions by linking self-determination to a "realistic view of freedom . . . the inner capacity and outer opportunity to make reasoned choices among possible, socially acceptable alternatives" (Perlman, 1971, p. 144, as cited in Wesley, 1996, p. 119).

Consider the case of Dorothy, a woman who entered into a second marriage after being widowed for several years and became a victim of emotional abuse, sexual abuse, and financial exploitation. She had no children from her first marriage, but in her widowhood lived in an active community and had many friends. The man she met and married was a businessman from another state. After marrying they returned to his home. She merged her finances with his and her furniture and other items were incorporated into his house. In her new location she had no friends, or no family. Because she did not drive and public transportation was not available she soon became fully dependent upon her husband, and was isolated from the community. She was emotionally abused by her husband and his two adult children and soon realized that her new husband participated in sexual activities outside of their marriage. After about six months of marriage, he brought his sex circle home and demanded that she participate by being the "audience." She became severely depressed and had a few hospital admissions where medical social workers surmised something was wrong at home but did not file a report because she did not "admit" to anything. She refused all mental health intervention although she was diagnosed as clinically depressed. Eventually her mental state was such that she collapsed and became comatose during one of the sex parties. Her husband fearing she was dying called an ambulance. The Emergency Medical Team (EMT) witnessing her condition and suspicious of the husband's demeanor made a referral to protective services (Author case file[1]). Why did the EMT report his suspicions to APS and the medical social workers, although they suspected an abusive situation, did not?

Phillips and Rempusheski (1986) examined this question citing problems with case detection and the lack of skills of health professions in reading the signs of abuse and neglect. This study cited one health respondent stating that "there's no rule written that all of a sudden, this is an abuse case. Some people may say that something is abusive but there's a whole other side to it (SW104)" (Phillips and Rempusheski, 1986, 135-136). This study also cited the justification used by health workers: the client's right-to-choose. "That's one thing working with the elderly; they have the right to choose. Sometimes they make real bad decisions but as long as they are able they can choose (SW104)" (Phillips and Rempusheski, 1986, 137). At what point is a depressed, or sick, or abused person unable to choose?

The theory of learned helplessness may explain why months or years of abuse, or neglect, or being financially exploited would leave a victim feeling that his or her situation was not solvable, even by a trained professional. Depressed people and most victims of abuse suffer from some level of depression, thus they may be indecisive, or lack the ability to make any decision beyond what to eat or when to bathe or go to bed. Poor client motivation resulting from depression may make the simplest change seem insurmountable. The relationship the victim shares with the perpetrator, as well as the developing relationship with the professional, may present a host of feelings for the victim inhibiting him or her to act on one's own behalf. At what point does a professional disregard a victim's refusal for intervention and assert some authority to protect the individual from further harm, at the very least by filing a report of suspected abuse or neglect?

I asked Dorothy two years after APS had intervened if her right to self-determination superseded the intervention she received. By then she had obtained a divorce and was relocated to her own apartment in an elderly complex. Her response was quite direct and clear. "How dare you professionals speak of self-determination when I was obviously suffering?" She explained that she was incapable of telling anyone about the abuse as it was happening because of her feelings of shame and that the abuse was her fault for marrying him. She also stated she could not effectively evaluate choices offered because she did not feel she deserved anything more than what she was getting from her husband. She said her isolation greatly impacted her perspective and that what she needed was immediate distancing from her situation, at least initially, before she could effectively make her own decisions (Author case files). How do professionals recognize when a client has compromised decision-making and is in need of professional direction?

THE PROFESSIONAL ROLE IN CLIENT DECISION-MAKING

The very contact with a professional may impact the decisional ability of the older person, especially an APS worker who is uninvited by the victim and often visiting the alleged victim within his or her own home. Such clients are involuntary and "Social work practice tends to ignore involuntary interactions since most social work techniques assume that the client has the right of self-determination" (Hasenfeld, 1987, 474). How does APS training integrate the notion of the involuntary client with their intervention strategies? The older person's attitude about the APS worker visiting him or her, the allegations being investigated, and the APS worker's approach with the alleged victim will greatly impact the victim's decision-making. For example, I work with many older people who compromise their own health because they do not want to complain about how they are feeling or how the prescribed drugs make them feel to the "busy" doctor. These clients see medical doctors as having an authority over them and better able to assess their bodies' needs than they are able to do. They tend then to expect direction instead of entering into a mutual problem-solving relationship. If some victims of elder abuse perceive the APS worker as having authority to solve the abuse, might these victims be waiting for direction to resolve their immediate situations thereby undervaluing their own role in problem-solving?

The reason for the professional-client exchange, whether initiated by the client or mandated by a report, will affect the developing professional relationship. It is in the context of this relationship that clients give information about themselves and their families, ask necessary questions, weigh the suggested alternatives, build the needed trust, and develop the confidence that this specific professional has the skill, the interest, the knowledge and the means to help them. In abuse situations where often trust between the elder and a family member, who is usually the perpetrator of abuse, has been violated, trusting an unknown professional may be difficult indeed. Furthermore, it is unlikely that anyone, once they have entered into a relationship, can autonomously decide anything. Within any relationship, voluntarily or involuntarily, one ceases being totally autonomous and is influenced by the exchange. Part of the process then of determining a client's decision-making ability is found first in the establishment of a solid client-worker relationship, and the establishment of rapport begins with the professional. Consider this APS worker's view of building a relationship when attempting to intervene: "Experience teaches you how to be a salesman for services to clients who don't think they want them, but who clearly need them . . . I work real hard to sell myself [to the client]" (Bergeron, 1998, 218). What happens then if a professional has good knowledge but cannot effectively build relationships with an elder victim? Is it possible that a client might refuse services, or not appropriately hear solutions to his or her situation offered by the APS worker because of an impaired relationship? Does that affect the client's ability to make difficult decisions about the abusive situation, thereby affecting his or her ability to self-determine?

Additionally, the decision-making ability of the client may partially rest on the "clinical observation, inference, reasoning, and judgment of the social worker" (Nurius & Gibson, 1990). How a worker interprets what is being said, or not being said, by the client will impact the interview and the assessment, the intervention, and the clinical judgments. The client's ability to make decisions cannot be viewed only from the standpoint of the client, but must consider whether the professional engaged with the client has understood what the client has shared. What if the elderly client has a personality disorder that further inhibits the forming of a relationship (Rose, Soares, & Joseph, 1993) causing the professional to prematurely disengage? Or what if the APS worker does not properly interpret the culturally laden responses of the abused victim? An abused victim's refusal-for-services may not necessarily mean the victim does not want to be helped but may reflect factors of an impaired professional relationship, or lack of the professional's training.

The authority or lack of authority of the professional also affects how clients make decisions. Authority may promote decisions not really desired by the client or it may give clients the strength to make decisions they find extremely difficult and risk-filled. The agency also influences the client's decisional process because of the agency's power to influence its workers to problem-solve with all clients or to only problem-solve with selected clients (e.g., the terms "motivated" or "compliant" assigned to clients), thus affecting the professional engagement process. If elder victims "refuse" services, does the culture of the responding agency "accept" that as a means of balancing high caseloads, or minimal community services, or inadequate funding? One APS worker expressed concern about this issue saying,

> Well, I've always said that social work is a job in which the State pays you money to be an advocate for the client to get the client services that the State really doesn't want to pay for them to have. (Bergeron, 1998, 216)

SELF-DETERMINATION AND THE NOTION OF CHOICE

The notion of choice is paramount if one is to self-determine. Victims need to know and understand the range of choice available to remedy their situation before being able to self-determine. Conversely the alternatives given to victims need to be of more than one alternative and must represent a range of choice reflective of the victim's community, culture, and philosophy-of-life. Too frequently a nursing home is the only alternative or solution given to severe victims of elder abuse and neglect, and because many victims would rather be abused or neglected than go to a nursing home (Wolf & Pillemer, 1989) this is an inappropriate choice inhibiting one's ability to self-determine. Victims need to see alternatives that mirror healthier versions of their current situations, producing a sense of comfort or security and hope that things may change without their losing the very foundation of their life-style and life-choices.

For example, in the aforementioned hoarding case of Fannie Claussen, she apparently agreed to go to a hotel room but left after one night to return to living in her yard. I would surmise the choice of a hotel room was a poor alternative to offer a woman who loved animals and "stuff." Hotel rooms are generally neat, clean, orderly, disengaging. What would someone like Ms. Claussen *do* in such a space? Where would she find her comfort zone to encourage her to allow professionals to change her home space? Ms. Claussen needed a foster home with people she could relate to and that afforded a connection to her neighborhood, a place with clutter and lived-in space. She needed to visually see what her life could be like if she allowed professionals to intervene. Under the best of circumstances people tend to make decisions that produce the least amount of change because change is hard. Abused victims need choices that still connect them to the familiar. Attention must be given to the least disruptive alternatives to victims. Respect for the victim's life-style and philosophy about living should be part of every alternative that is reasonably possible. Currently the services for abused and neglected elderly victims are narrowly defined by those services for frail health-impaired elders. When clients refuse intervention are they self-determining that they do not want to change their situation, or that they find the alternatives offered insufficient for their needs?

CLIENT COMPETENCY AND CAPACITY

Lack of victim competency justifies enacting protective services regardless of the victim desires. However, even in cases of client incompetence, practitioners are to act with the least restrictive measures in accordance with what is known about the values of the victim. This presents a real dilemma to APS workers. Is it sufficient to say that one is either competent or not competent? Or is it more reasonable to say that people have varying levels of competency dependent upon what is being decided? By what standards does one judge competency? Mini mental status exams may give professionals an indication that a victim is having difficulty processing information, or may give no indication at all. Certainly using trained professionals to administer an in-depth examination makes sense when a victim is in a precarious situation. But such exams are not always feasible because the victim may refuse to go to a clinic or professional office; professionals may not make house calls, or may not be locally available, particularly in rural settings. APS agencies may not have a budget to pay for competency exams. Furthermore, accurate results may be compromised if not given over a period of appointments and if administered at either the "best" or the "worst" functioning time of the victim. Professionals working in elder abuse tend to prefer the term capacity because it may allow for a more concrete means of assessing what someone is capable of accomplishing, under what conditions, and what decisions tend to confound the victim's task accomplishment.

Along with the prior concepts of life style and philosophies of life, some of the factors needing consideration are one's past capacity to make decisions, the history of relationships reflective in the abusive relationship, and health issues.

Past History of and Current Decisional Abilities

When interviewing an older person a complexity of issues exists that requires skilled observation and skilled interviewing. Often older people take longer to engage than do younger people because of cultural norms about sharing private matters. Older people may be less accepting of interventions by agencies, particularly a government agency, than are younger people. Older people in rural settings may be more suspicious of formal systems than are their city-dwelling counterparts who have had more opportunity to experience them. Older people may also take longer to make decisions because they consider more than just their personal safety issue–which tends to be the only focus of APS workers. For example, concern for the perpetrator is not a consideration in APS laws, although by meeting the needs of the perpetrator (e.g., housing) in certain situations the abuse of the elder may be eliminated.

Elder abuse victims are often isolated. Sometimes this isolation is societal driven through retirement, changes in housing or relocation, reconfiguration of neighborhoods, or ageist policies and cultural attitudes. Sometimes it results from changing health status that makes the elderly person more homebound or removes informal networks by illness and death. Other times it may be the existence of long-time health or mental health issues. Isolation may be perpetrator driven, meaning the abuser isolates the victim from friends, family, and health professionals for control and to thwart abuse detection. Isolation over time may impede the ability to be flexible in thinking about alternatives to solve problems, particularly if coupled with depression.

Typically APS workers see abused and neglected elderly victims in crisis and after the abuse has been ongoing. This is because victims seldom self-refer, so most reports are made by a third party becoming aware of the abusive situation. Many times it is injury (e.g., a fractured hip) or a health issue (e.g., dehydration) that brings the victim into the healthcare system. Sick people have a harder time making decisions than do healthy people, and illness and institutionalization may add to the feelings of being in crisis and not in control. Making decisions when one is sick and in crisis is very difficult without proper support and elderly victims often lack strong, local supportive networks, which of course is one reason why they become victims.

If one is isolated, depressed, sick, and in crisis is it reasonable to expect that person to self-determine about the very situation of abuse that resulted in his or her current predicament? The types of decisions required of abuse victims go beyond the simple decisions of what to eat, what to wear, or when to go to bed. Abuse victims are often asked to "tell on" family members, or reveal financial scams or financial exploitation they find embarrassing, or to describe degrading treatment. They are then asked to self-determine with a professional a course-of-action to ameliorate the abuse or neglect. Such decision-making re-quires complex thinking of victims to separate themselves emotionally from their perpetrator, or to complete hierarchical choices way beyond their estab-lished routine–and often times the decisions they make will have conse-quences for the perpetrator, many of whom are their family members.

The types of decisions made throughout one's life also affects one's ability to self-determine and to make competent decisions. Good decision making takes practice. If people are told throughout their lives how to manage their af-fairs, their decisional skills will be impaired. If the elder's cultural background has been authority driven by family or the community, self-determination will not be feasible from an individual perspective. These victims may need strong guidance throughout the decisional process. Every APS worker should ask victims of elder abuse and neglect how decisions are routinely made within their families and who makes them.

An individual's locus of control is important in decision-making. Do vic-tims see that their decisions will influence their environment, thereby having an internal locus of control? Or do victims experience the environment and people as controlling them, thereby having an external locus of control? If one's belief is that decisions come from outside of one, is it reasonable to ex-pect that person to have the capacity to self-determine from an individual per-spective?

Family Relationships and Culture

Carol, an active 62-year-old woman, cared for her 85-year-old father. She sought services for her caregiving role. On her third agency visit the worker questioned her about a scarf fashionably tied around her neck but looking somewhat out of place in the warm weather, whereupon Carol broke down into tears. After a sensitive assessment it was discovered she was being repeat-edly strangled and raped by her 79-year-old uncle. This abuse began when she was 13-years-old and ended only when at 18-years-old she left for college and moved out-of-state. The abuse resumed immediately upon her return home to care for her ailing father who, in his demented state, offered her no protection. The scarf covered the bruising from repeated strangulations she endured (Au-thor case files).

If the abuse or neglect is perpetrated by a family member, the elder's deci-sion-making ability may be compromised not just because of feelings of fear, or guilt that these occurrences are his or her own fault, but also due to an alle-giance to the perpetrator. In the case of Carol, the power she gave her uncle was unrealistic given her current age and health and that of her uncle's. When the abuse began again she reacted as she did as an adolescent–powerless and resigned that she could not resist him. Furthermore, she had strong feelings of family pride and allegiance preventing her from risking the family's "good name" by taking action. Her commitment to the family's reputation and her perception of the status of her family within the community superseded her need of safety. And although she was competent in every other aspect of her life and was making good decisions for the provision of care to her father, she was incapable of thinking of alternatives for her own safety, or initially accepting service offered to end the abuse.

Older people abused by their adult children often have to let go of the deep felt obligation of parental care and duties before they can decide their own safety issues. If the abuse occurs because their children are developmentally disabled or have mental health issues, older people may refuse needed respite services for fear the abuse will be found out, or they may fail to seek help for fear of losing control of the fate of their disabled child. Unless these victims of abuse can be reassured that their child will not only have care, but be loved, they may be unable to "think beyond" that concern.

Victims whose adult children or other relatives abuse them because of substance abuse problems, or dependency for needed resources (e.g., money, food, shelter), may not admit to abuse for fear that criminal charges will be brought against the perpetrator to whom they still feel a deep sense of obligation. These victims' decision-making abilities may be compromised because they fear their child, or because they fear being abandoned by their child. Such victims may be concerned that they will be in a worse situation if their child is removed from their household. In the United States in-home health and community care supplements, not replaces, the care provided by families. Few communities can offer enough in-home services without additional family support; therefore it is very reasonable for older people to question where help will come from, particularly in rural areas, should their child leave the home. Victims may be concerned about who will provide weekend and holiday assistance, or evening help, or when the electricity and heat are lost during a blizzard. In the words of one man who suffered occasional beatings by his alcoholic son, "I have to measure my options. These [the beatings] don't happen very often. And he tries hard when he's not drunk. He takes care of the house; he fixes the windows, mows the grass. He makes sure there is food in the house . . . he's here at night. I couldn't stay here if he left" (Author case files).

Victims in abusive marriages may have many reasons for not seeking or refusing offers of help. Their shame about the situation, particularly if the victim is a man, and doubt about being believed, may limit their decisional process. Elder victims may be concerned about burdening their adult children with the healthcare needs of the spousal perpetrator or may view their children's needs above their own. If the spousal perpetrator also victimized the children when they were growing up, the spousal victim may hesitate in seeking their children's assistance. Felt obligation to marital vows and commitment to one's religious beliefs about such vows may impede rational choice for personal safety.

Health Issues

Abuse or neglect may exacerbate health conditions that compromise one's ability to effectively decide, e.g., lack of sleep, lack of food, dehydration, or improper medication or medical care, or mental health issues. McCreadie states that

> Mental and emotional problems may be both a cause and an effect of elder abuse. It would hardly be surprising if people living with abuse, some of which may be long term, displayed psychological effects. (1996a, p. 43, cited in Penhale and Kingston, 1995, 300)

Depression, discussed earlier, is certainly an inhibitor to decision-making. But so are other mental health issues. For example, hoarding behaviors like the case of Fannie Claussen, may be reflective of an obsessive-compulsive disorder (Thomas, 1997), thereby making it nearly impossible for the individual to decide on the necessary actions to resolve the hoarding behaviors. Sleep deprivation caused by super vigilance or unmanaged pain or lack of medical care will cause disorientation and impede a rational choice process.

SELF-DETERMINATION AND LEGAL RESPONSES

Respect for self-determination does not excuse the APS worker or other professionals from understanding legal remedies to difficult situations. In fact, the Code of Ethics (NASW, 2000) outlines the social worker's responsibility to seek support from other professionals if it is in the best interest of the client. Therefore, should the victim refuse intervention to ensure reasonable safety, the APS worker may need to explore legal remedies and, depending upon the legal response, the APS worker may need to invoke legal action without the client's permission.

Just as every state has some form of elder abuse protection law, every state also has protective order legislation for domestic abuse (Jordan, 2001). Such statutes offer protection based on the type of relationship between the victim and the perpetrator (e.g., by blood, marriage, adoption, and cohabitation). And some states go further by also recognizing dating couples and vulnerable adults as part of their statute (Jordan, 2001). All statutes require proof that abuse occurred (Jordan, 2001). Thus, protective order statutes may provide emergency and ongoing intervention if domestic violence can be proved. Such orders may give elderly victims protection from an abuser by minimizing, restricting, or eliminating their contact with one another. They may also provide temporary or ongoing financial support if it is established that there is a duty of the perpetrator to support the victim (typically husband or wife relationships) (Jordan, 2001). In addition, if a protective order is carefully and thoughtfully written it may be tailored to meet some of the individual abusive behaviors of the perpetrator, e.g., stating the perpetrator cannot have access to the victim's mail (Jordan, 2001). This may afford the victim with necessary protection and enough distance from the perpetrator to eventually allow the victim to gain insight for future decisions.

Making a report to APS services, and an APS worker responding to a case of elder abuse, does not preclude a simultaneous referral for domestic violence to help in protecting the victim. Nor does it prevent the APS worker from making such a referral in responding to the abuse report. Many APS agencies are now working closely with advocates of domestic violence to develop a team approach and alternatives for elder domestic abuse victims. These teams may assess an intervention course-of-action should the victim by his or her refusal for an APS intervention remain in grave danger.

Criminal courts may be useful for both crimes to the person (e.g., physical and sexual abuse and domestic violence) and crimes involving property (theft, credit card fraud, forgery, etc.) (Jordan, 2001). APS workers need to work in conjunction with attorneys and law enforcement when certain cases show criminal activity, even if the perpetrator is a family member. However, family dynamics are complex and proving undue influence may be difficult. Additionally, due to cognitive changes in the elder or feelings of obligation toward the perpetrator, elders may be poor witnesses. Consequently, careful consideration must be given if the filing of charges represents a reasonable solution or will further compromise the elder. Rein issues this warning about using the legal and criminal system:

> . . . the focus of our present approach [of the legal system]–which often evaluates the candidate for intervention without also requiring official evaluation of the programs, motives, interests, and moral claims of the proposed intervenors–is dangerously narrow and may produce substantial harm [to the ward]. (1992, p. 1821)

Rein's concern provides a caution about the rigidity of the legal system, which should be taken very seriously. Once invoked, the individual's right to self-determine ceases and mediation among family members may be impaired. But this warning also speaks to the need to develop community or consulting teams that include legal and law expertise that may help decide which cases would most successfully be resolved using criminal intervention. Furthermore, sometimes just the introduction of law enforcement will act as an intervention by motivating the perpetrator to stop the abuse or by motivating the victim to utilize a non-criminal solution (e.g., removing money management from the victim may stop the financial exploitation).

Power-of-attorney (POA), conservatorships, and guardianships are all legal devices that may be suggested or petitioned for if victims are incapable of decision-making. For example, if an older person is self-neglecting because he does not want to pay his bills, yet he has adequate funds to do so, he may grant a POA to someone to pay only those bills necessary to meet his basic living needs (Jordan, 2001). But deciding which clients should have such devices is often difficult, or not supported by the intervening APS agency. Additionally, because it is relatively easy to execute and abuse a POA it is imperative that great thought be given to the selection process of the agent and the subsequent accounting process. Abused and neglected elders may be without appropriate family members to act as agents and many communities may not have a formal system (such as a Guardianship Program, or Representative Payee Project) to provide ethical decision-makers. Conservatorships may be given over property and may be useful in resolving dramatic cases of hoarding. Guardianships may be given over either person or property, or may include both, and can be extremely useful in providing an advocate who can monitor the victim's situation and enforce actions to prevent or minimize future abuse and neglect. Yet, traditionally APS workers have been hesitant about and, in some states, discouraged from utilizing the legal system, in part due to a fear of minimizing the victim's right to self-determine. Although there needs to be a judicial selection of appropriate cases with careful consideration for the appropriate legal device and surrogate decision-maker, the APS worker's difficulty in deciding what cases merit such referrals does not justify discounting legal devices as legitimate tools for practice.

The use of law enforcement is still developing in the field of elder protection work. Traditionally, crimes committed within one's home against another family member have been viewed differently than crimes committed by strangers. Thus, the Justice Department has recognized that domestic violence needs different solutions than typical street crimes. Allowing families to work with approved human service agencies to resolve issues of violence and preserve the family unit has been one goal in enacting protection laws. The criminal system is not well understood by the general public and once invoked personal choice is eliminated. Yet, invoking law enforcement may not be a choice of the victim or the APS worker if a crime has been committed. Heisler asserts that "In serious cases, the criminal justice system may provide the only way to protect the vulnerable elder" (1991, p. 25). When then does a professional seek counsel, against the will of the victim, to introduce legal devices, or begin a criminal investigation? By doing so does the APS worker violate the client's right to self-determine? How does the notion of liberty and justice relate to the professional ethics of helping?

CONCLUSION

Professionals entrusted with the duty-to-protect victims of elder abuse absolutely cannot use the principle of self-determination as the primary reason to leave elder victims in life-threatening situations, or to unconditionally accept victims' refusal-for-services. Too many factors mitigate individual choice in life-threatening situations whether the abuse or neglect is in the privacy of one's home or is in the full view of the community. Professionals need to apply critical thinking considering the political, social and environmental factors that go beyond only the victim (Gambrill, 1990). Without consideration of culture and community, including the responsibility of the victim to the community, determinations to intervene in elder abuse may be grossly miscalculated by the worker. Gambrill warns that "[The] decisions to intervene [by the social worker] may be made when there is no justifiable reason to do so, [or] a decision may be made not to intervene when intervention would help clients to enhance the quality of their lives . . ." (1990, p. 20). Thus, professional examination of how to work with elder victims of abuse refusing services must be paramount in the elder protection field. Honoring client choice may not necessarily mean honoring the overt refusal for intervention. Moody (1988) suggests that when professionals accept clients' refusal-for-services that it ". . . may be little different from patient abandonment . . ."–a clear violation of a social worker's professional Ethical Code. Instead he suggests the notion of "negotiated consent." This would equate to practitioners offering degrees of assistance that minimize the abuse and provide reasonable relief for the victim, or that provide assistance to the perpetrator to resolve conditions that may trigger abusive behavior. Choices may need to include safety training for victims and living alternative choices that match the victim's life style and capacity for self-care, or providing housing assistance to remove abusive relatives. The challenge, of course, is to find and create those alternatives that reflect a range from a minimal safety net to the maximum safety net for the victim. Legal systems need to carefully weigh their criticisms of a system that has been supported by laws to protect elders but has received little funding to develop appropriate resources or direction to do so. Researchers and practitioners must study the role of self-determination as perceived by clients who have successfully resolved severe abuse and neglect.

The right to decide direction of one's life is very important and cannot be minimized. But, so, too, is the mutual responsibility of the individual to the community and the professional's duty to promote the safety of elders suffering from gross abuse and neglect. This responsibility and duty demands as much attention as does respecting one's right-to-choose. This article provides only a cursory examination of elder abuse and self-determination. Self-determination in elder protection work is in great need of research and debate. Cases where abuse and neglect have been reduced or eliminated are ideal to retrospectively interview those victims about their ability to problem solve and their expectations of professionals who assisted them. Laws that only allow for investigating and substantiating allegations of abuse, but then allow exclusive rights to the victim to remain in serious, life-threatening situations because of his or her "right to choose" begs our immediate attention. It also threatens our humanity as professionals and as people living in the same community with elder victims of maltreatment.

Understanding all the factors that may impede rational choice is complex and requires highly sophisticated and critical thinking. Professionals working with the elderly and APS workers must procure on-going training, consultation and supervision, and participate in collaborative activities regarding the principle of self-determination and the duty-to-protect abused elders. In answering the question: "Do we know enough?" given what was presented here, and all I wish space and time would have allowed me to add, we do not. The next question is "Are we willing to learn?"

NOTE

1. Author case files: Client names and other key information have been changed to protect confidentiality.

REFERENCES

Bergeron, L. R. (1998). Identification of the decisional factors used by adult protective service workers when intervening in cases of elder physical abuse. UMI Dissertation Abstracts, 9828039 (Doctoral Dissertation, Boston College, 1997). *http://www.umi.com.*

Bergeron, L. R. (1999). Decision-making and adult protective services workers: Identifying critical factors. *Journal of Elder Abuse & Neglect, 10* (3/4), 87-113.

Bergeron, L. R. (2003). Elder abuse: Clinical assessment & obligation to report. In K. Kendall-Tackett (Ed.), *Health Consequences of Abuse in the Family: A Clinical Guide for Evidence-Based Practice* (pp. 109-128). Washington, DC: American Psychological Association.

Burchell, J., & Swedlund, E. (2004, June 23). She leaves blessed mess, for now. *Arizona Daily Star. http://www.dailystar.com/dailystar/printDS/27201.php.* Retrieved June 25, 2004.

Callahan, J. (1997). Assisted suicide, community, and the common good. *Health & Social Work, 22* (4), 243-246.

Ewalt, P., & Mokuau, N. (1995). Self-determination from a Pacific perspective. *Social Work, 40* (2), 168-175.

Gambrill, E. (1990). *Critical Thinking in Clinical Practice.* San Francisco, CA: Jossey-Bass.

Ganzini, L., Lee, M., Heintz, R., & Bloom, J. (1993). Is the patient self-determination act appropriate for elderly persons hospitalized for depression? *The Journal of Clinical Ethics, 4*(1), 46-50.

Hancock, L. (2004, June 13). Judge, lawyer fight elder neglect: Cases show agency did little to fix elderly's deplorable conditions. *The Dallas Morning News. http://www.dallasnews.com/cgi-bin/gold_print.cgi.* Retrieved June 25, 2004.

Hasenfeld, Y. (1987). Power in social work practice. *Social Service Review, 61* (3), 469-483.

Heisler, C. (1991). The role of the criminal justice system in elder abuse cases. *Journal of Elder Abuse & Neglect, 3* (1), 5-33.

Jordan, L. (2001). Elder abuse and domestic violence: Overlapping issues and legal remedies. *American Journal of Family Law, 15,* 147-157.

Mixson, P. (1995). An adult protective services perspective. *Journal of Elder Abuse & Neglect, 7*(2/3), 69-87.

Moody, H. (1988). From informed consent to negotiated consent. *The Gerontologist, 28*(suppl.), 64-70.

NASW (National Association of Social Workers). (2000). *Code of Ethics of the National Association of Social Workers.* Washington, DC: Author.

National Adult Protective Services Association. (2004). *Ethical Principles and Best Practice Guidelines.* Boulder, CO: Author.

Nurius, P., & Gibson, J. (June, 1990). Clinical observation, inference, reasoning, and judgment in social work: An update. *Social Work Research & Abstracts,* 18-25.

Penhale, B., & Kingston, P. (1997). Elder abuse, mental health, and later life: Steps toward an understanding. *Aging & Mental Health, 1* (4), 296-304.

Phillips, L., & Rempusheski, V. (1986). Making decisions about elder abuse. *The Journal of Contemporary Social Work,* March, 131-140.

Rein, J. (1992). Preserving dignity and self-determination of the elderly in the face of competing interests and grim alternatives: A proposal for statutory refocus and reform. *The George Law Review, 60* (6), 1818-1887.

Rose, M., Soares, H., & Joseph, C. (1993). Frail elderly clients with personality disorders: A challenge for social work. *Journal of Gerontological Social Work, 19* (3/4), 153-165.

Simon, M. L. (1992). *An Exploratory Study of Adult Protective Service Programs; Repeat Elder Abuse Clients.* AARP: Washington, DC.

St. James, P. (2001). Challenges in elder mistreatment programs and policy. *Journal of Gerontological Social Work, 36* (3/4), 127-140.

Thomas, N. (1997). Hoarding: Eccentricity or pathology: When to intervene? *Journal of Gerontological Social Work, 29* (1), 45-55.

Wesley, C. (1996). Social work and end-of-life decisions: Self-determination and the common good. *Health & Social Work, 21* (2), 115-122.

Wolf, R., & Pillemer, K. (1989) *Helping Elderly Victims: The Reality of Elder Abuse.* New York: Columbia University Press.

Use of a Single Page
Elder Abuse Assessment
and Management Tool:
A Practical Clinician's Approach
to Identifying Elder Mistreatment

Patricia A. Bomba, MD, FACP

SUMMARY. Elder abuse is a growing, alarming public health issue. As health care professionals, our challenge is to balance our duty to protect the safety of the vulnerable elder with the elder's right to self-determination. Clinicians in busy practice settings across the continuum of care as well as community-based social workers, emergency medical system, police, and banking personnel are collaborative partners needing tools that focus on early recognition, assessment, intervention, and management of elder abuse. A simple one-page tool that provides principles of assessment and management, best practice guidelines and screening questions will hopefully serve to raise awareness of this important public health issue and maintain a high index of suspicion for elder abuse, neglect and financial exploitation. *[Article copies available for a fee from The Haworth Document Delivery Service: 1-800-HAWORTH. E-mail address: <docdelivery@haworthpress.com> Website: <http://www.HaworthPress.com> © 2006 by The Haworth Press, Inc. All rights reserved.]*

[Haworth co-indexing entry note]: "Use of a Single Page Elder Abuse Assessment and Management Tool: A Practical Clinician's Approach to Identifying Elder Mistreatment." Bomba, Patricia A. Co-published simultaneously in *Journal of Gerontological Social Work* (The Haworth Press, Inc.) Vol. 46, No. 3/4, 2006, pp. 103-122 ; and: *Elder Abuse and Mistreatment: Policy, Practice, and Research* (ed: M. Joanna Mellor, and Patricia Brownell) The Haworth Press, Inc., 2006, pp. 103-122. Single or multiple copies of this article are available for a fee from The Haworth Document Delivery Service [1-800-HAWORTH, 9:00 a.m. - 5:00 p.m. (EST). E-mail address: docdelivery@haworthpress.com].

Available online at http://www.haworthpress.com/web/JGSW
© 2006 by The Haworth Press, Inc. All rights reserved.
doi:10.1300/J083v46n03_06

KEYWORDS. Elder abuse, neglect, tools, guidelines, screening, geriatric syndrome

INTRODUCTION

Elder abuse is a growing, alarming public health issue resulting in personal and healthcare costs for victims as well as the health care system. It is an independent risk factor that increases mortality rates in older adults (Lachs, 1998). Elder abuse is multidimensional, includes acts of commission as well as omission, and involves medical, psychological, social, legal, ethical, financial, and environmental issues.

Health care professionals are in a unique position to identify and intervene on behalf of their patients. To do so, all health care professionals must maintain a high index of suspicion for elder abuse, neglect, and financial exploitation in all settings across the continuum of care. In addition to considering elder abuse and neglect as a possibility, the physician must commit to brief, rapid, reliable screenings of all elders, understand how to perform more detailed diagnostic assessments when needed, including capacity assessment, and utilize a consistent approach to management and monitoring. To assure effective integration and coordination, all professionals must be prepared to work as part of an interdisciplinary team. Physicians, nurses, and social workers alike must recognize when to refer patients for additional assessment from colleagues and when and how to use community resources effectively.

Elder abuse is a problem in every community and among all social strata. It is underrecognized, underreported, and underprosecuted. Social workers who work primarily in the community and outside health care systems play a significant role in identifying elder abuse and neglect. It is critical that elder mistreatment is considered among their senior center members, senior housing residents, community center members, employee assistance program clients, and all venues where they come in contact with seniors, their caregivers and potential perpetrators. A high index of suspicion leads to early recognition and identification. Understanding the need and when to integrate with the physician and appropriate community resources is critical.

As health care professionals, our challenge is to balance our duty to protect the safety of the vulnerable elder with the elder's right to self-determination. For clinicians in busy practices, a simple one-page tool that provides principles of assessment and management, best practice guidelines and screening questions will hopefully also serve to raise awareness of this important public health issue and maintain a high index of suspicion for elder abuse, neglect, and financial exploitation. This is true in all settings across the continuum of care. Community-based social workers, as well as emergency medical system, police, and banking personnel and all citizens are partners needing tools that focus on early recognition, assessment, intervention, and use of appropriate resources.

If we are to create lasting system solutions for this major public health issue, action must take place on the medical, psychological, social, and legal levels and care must be carefully coordinated among multiple systems. For healthcare professionals, the cases are demanding and often frustrating. For older adults, solutions are difficult and frequently unacceptable. In the next twenty years when the population of seniors has doubled, the problem of elder abuse will become more serious if steps are not taken now to address the problem. The pain and suffering, the loss of trust and loss of resources experienced by seniors will be matched by a significant cost to the government and to society as a whole. We clearly need a national elder abuse strategy. For the present, part of the solution lies in framing elder abuse as a geriatric syndrome, utilizing an interdisciplinary approach integrating community resources, developing an evidence base through rigorous research and in increasing professional and community awareness of this hidden epidemic.

If we are to create optimal solutions, we must recognize both the demographic variables as well as the diminishing social network and poor social functioning associated with signs of potential abuse. Characteristics of the older adult's cognitive, behavioral, and medical health, coupled with their functional capacity must be understood to help appreciate their vulnerability. Furthermore, given the demographics of aging, we must appreciate the burden of chronic disease in light of the trajectory of various chronic diseases, particularly with advancing chronic illness at the end-of-life. Effective palliative care must be provided.

As defined by the Institute of Medicine (Field & Cassel, 1997), palliative care is intended to seek to prevent, relieve, reduce, or soothe the symptoms of disease or disorder without an expectation of cure. Not only is palliative care in this broad sense not restricted to the dying or those receiving hospice services, it also focuses on the emotional, spiritual, and practical needs and goals of patients and their loved ones.

As defined by the Center for the Advancement of Palliative Care in 2002, palliative care is interdisciplinary in that it aims at ameliorating the suffering and improving the quality of life for patients with advanced illness. It is offered at the same time as other appropriate medical treatment, and includes support for families as well.

Raising awareness of elder abuse and palliative care among health care professionals is essential if we are to bridge the educational gaps that exist. Appropriate attention to both offers the opportunity to reduce suffering and improve the quality of life for our elders. It offers the professional the opportunity to make a difference in the life of an individual and to have that individual make a difference in their life by restoring a sense of professionalism.

BACKGROUND

Demographics of Aging, Chronic Diseases, and the End-of-Life

At the turn of the 20th Century, life expectancy for the average American was 47. By the turn of the 21st Century, life expectancy had improved to approximately 77-years-old (Center for Disease Control, 2003). This is primarily due to improved public health, sanitation, and improved healthcare. By the year 2030, twenty percent (20) of the American population, or 70 million people, will be over the age of 65 (Kaplan & Peres, 2002).

Currently there are 78 million baby boomers (people currently aged 39 to 57-years-old) representing 27.5 percent of the total population. By 2030, the baby boomers will be 66 to 84 years and are projected to comprise 20 percent of the total population. The senior population reached approximately 30 million in 1998, will reach almost 40 million by 2011 and 50 million by 2019 (Bureau of the Census, 1997). The fastest growing segment of the population includes those who are 85+, a cohort with the highest prevalence rates of dementia.

With this improved life expectancy, the incidence of chronic disease has increased. Chronic diseases are among the most prevalent, costly, and potentially preventable of all health problems. Approximately 80% of persons 65 or older nationally have at least one chronic condition, and 50% have at least two. In addition, there is an increasing prevalence of chronic disease that is expected to rise with time (Center to Advance Palliative Care, 2002). While clinical advances have reduced the effects of many chronic diseases, our society has been unsuccessful in changing the behaviors that cause or exacerbate these diseases. Obesity, a preventable risk factor for chronic diseases such as diabetes, cardiovascular disease, cancer and stroke, is now epidemic. Nationally, almost 75% of adults 55- to 64-years-old are 'overweight' or 'obese' (Fitch, Pyenson, Abbs, & Liang, 2004; Finger Lakes Health Systems Agency, 2004).

Advances in medicine and technology have allowed more and more Americans to live longer with chronic and advanced chronic illness. Patients with chronic disease often suffer from pain and depression, which further complicates their management. Furthermore, there is variation in the decline in function and health status as well as variation in progression of the expected course of different chronic diseases (EPEC, 2005). In particular in the elderly, often multiple chronic diseases coexist, adding to the complexity of disease and care management and the potential for abuse and neglect.

Caring for seniors, particularly at the end-of-life, has also changed dramatically in recent years as life expectancies have increased, chronic disease rates have risen, and families, the health care systems, and society have changed.

There has been a marked shift in values in our society. We value productivity, youth, and independence while devaluing age, family, and interdependent caring for one another.

Without increased awareness of the issue and attention to care and coordination of health, social, legal and human services, one can expect the prevalence of elder abuse and neglect to increase. As technology has advanced, death has become viewed by society as "failure" and "optional." Since the majority of the 2.4 million Americans that die each year are aged 65 or above and since death is an inevitable part of aging, one can expect the demand for end-of-life care to continue to increase as the population demographics shift. While expertise in palliation of pain and symptoms at the end of life has been developed, palliative care has not been well integrated with management of chronic diseases or incorporated into the continuum of medical management from health and wellness to the end-of-life. Failure to provide palliative care to our seniors is the ultimate form of elder abuse.

Elder Mistreatment

Elder abuse is an all-inclusive term representing all types of mistreatment or abusive behavior towards older adults. This may be an act of commission or abuse or an act of omission or neglect. It may be intentional or unintentional. Whether a behavior can be labeled as abusive, neglectful, or exploitive depends on its frequency, duration, intensity, severity, consequences, and cultural context. In my clinical discussions with older adults, I have found that the term mistreatment was preferred.

There are several types of elder abuse, including physical, psychological, sexual, or financial exploitation. It also includes self-neglect, abandonment, and domestic violence of late life. Neglect is the most prevalent form of elder abuse while financial exploitation is the fastest growing form and is frequently linked with other types of abuse.

Definitions and legal terminology varies from state to state. As defined by the National Center on Elder Abuse (2005), physical abuse is the use of physical force that results in injury, physical pain, or impairment. Sexual abuse is defined as nonconsensual sexual contact of any kind with an elderly person. Psychological abuse is defined as the infliction of anguish, pain, or distress through verbal or nonverbal acts. Neglect is defined as the refusal or failure to fulfill any part of a person's obligations or duties to an elder. Abandonment is defined as the desertion of an elderly person by an individual who has assumed responsibility for providing care for an elder, or by a person with physical custody of an elder. Financial exploitation is defined as the illegal or improper use of an elder's funds, property, or assets. It is also recognized that victims of domestic violence grow old.

PUBLIC HEALTH ISSUE

Incidence and Prevalence

Elder abuse occurs in both domestic and institutional settings. In the preceding decade, five community surveys were done that show 4-6% of older adults report experiencing instances of domestic elder abuse, neglect, and financial exploitation.

In order to obtain more valid incidence data, Congress mandated a national study in 1996. A "sentinel" approach was employed, similar to previous federally sponsored child abuse surveys. This assumes that reported cases present only the proverbial "tip of the iceberg" and that many more cases in the community are never reported. Through a random sampling process, twenty counties were selected to service the sample sites. In each county, information on the cases was obtained from the local adult protective services agency and a specifically trained group of individuals, or the sentinels, who were drawn from agencies that normally serve older people such as hospitals and clinics and law enforcement agencies, senior citizens programs, and banking institutions.

The results of the National Elder Abuse Incidence Study (Tartara, Thomas et al., 1998) estimated that nearly half a million persons aged 60 and older living in domestic settings were abused, neglected or exploited in the United States in 1996. Of this total, only 70,942 cases were reported and substantiated by adult protective services. The remaining were not reported, but were identified by the "sentinels." That is to say that for every case reported to adult protective, it is assumed that five cases were not reported. Further projecting the estimates, but recognizing those that were never reported–it was estimated that there were between 820,000 and 1.86 million abused older people in the country.

The National Elder Abuse Incidence Study, which was published in 1998, found that the median age of the victims was 76.5 years and that elders 80 years of age and older were abused two to three times more often. Fifty percent of individuals were physically dependent on others. Females were abused more often than males, after accounting for their proportion in the aging population. Ninety percent of the time perpetrators were family members. The perpetrators often had a history of substance abuse. In addition, it found that of the most frequent reporters of Elder Abuse to Adult Protective Services were family members; hospitals were responsible for 17.3% of such reports, while physicians, nurses, and clinics in the community only reported about 8-10% of cases. Although Medicaid clients are more frequently reported as victims, it is because they have more contact with "social systems" and not because they are poor. It is estimated that the number of elder mistreatment cases will increase in the next several decades as the older population increases (National Research Council, 2003).

Mortality Rates

Elder Abuse results in unnecessary suffering, injury, pain, decreased quality of life, and loss or violation of human rights. Most importantly, it results in increased mortality rates (Lachs, 1998). Lachs evaluated data from the New England Established Population for Epidemiological Studies on the Elderly, which followed an annual heath survey of 2,812 community-dwelling adults who are 65 years of age or older. He compared this data against reports of elder abuse and neglect made to the local adult protective service over a 9-year period of time. The survival rates of the non-abused and abused were tracked. By the 13th year following the initiation of the study, 40% of the non-reported, that is, the non-abused or non-neglected, group was still alive, versus 17% of those seen for self-neglect, while only 9% of those seen for elder mistreatment were still living. These figures were adjusted to account for all possible factors that might affect mortality including age, gender, income, functional status, cognitive status, diagnosis, and social support. No other significant factors predictive of mortality were found. These findings are alarming and underscore the need for more research, not only on the psychosocial and physical consequences of mistreatment, but also on the effectiveness of current intervention strategies.

GERIATRIC SYNDROME

Given the aging demographics, the incidence of elder abuse and the impact on mortality rates, it is essential that all health care professionals have a consistent strategy in approaching the problem. To be effective, the generic unwillingness to address family violence in all forms as well as causes that are unique to elder abuse must be overcome. From the perspective of physicians, Lachs identified three major causes generic to the problem of family violence, namely, clinical and academic discomfort, time and reimbursement constraints, and perceived impotence (1995).

Many physicians may not feel comfortable inquiring with patients about domestic violence, nor feel clinically competent because they lack formal training. The same holds true for other health care professionals. Family violence does not fit neatly within the traditional medical paradigm of symptoms, diagnosis, and treatment. Furthermore, personal identification with patients might preclude the proper evaluation of family violence. From an academic perspective, we need additional evidence-based research focused on elder abuse and neglect. Although it is beginning to emerge, it is woefully behind child abuse and domestic violence.

Time and reimbursement constraints are repeatedly cited as major barriers. While it is true that proper evaluation of family violence and/or elder abuse is a time consuming process, a complete assessment may not be practical, particularly if this is discovered in the midst of routine evaluation. Appropriate counseling is difficult to perform in a 15-minute routine visit, especially if there is not a clear understanding of an approach to the problem. In addition, awareness of and relationships with available community resources provide professionals with an important timesaving advantage.

Sadly, many physicians perceive their inability to make a difference. In facilitated dialogue with physicians over the past three years, many have expressed their belief that it was the duty of the victims to separate themselves from an abusive environment and that they doubted that counseling was able to achieve a positive outcome. Nurses, social workers, and others in the field affirm this attitude. This too is likely the result of the lack of formal training. Many also expressed unsatisfactory outcomes with previous patients, which has created skepticism that they could serve any useful role. This further serves to have them view the problem as a social issue and outside their professional boundaries. Education and working in collaboration across professional lines provides health care professionals the opportunity to understand each other's professional viewpoint and language. If done consistently, in the long run, the patient and the professionals are all winners.

From a clinical perspective, ageism in medical practice is rather pervasive. Ageism refers to a tendency to dismiss many abnormal disease processes as normal aging. Similarly, signs and symptoms of elder abuse may be written off as inevitable, or ascribed to other diseases. Fractures can be attributed to osteoporosis. Direct reports of abuse may be dismissed as dementia, delirium, delusion, or confusion. Side effects of polypharmacy may be missed and ascribed to old age. Depression and pain may be underreported by the patient, unrecognized by the health care professional and undertreated by the physician. Since chronic pain can lead to depression and in turn social isolation and neglect, early identification is critical.

Failure to thrive is often blamed on general frailty, when in fact it can be the result of the deliberate withholding of food or medicines by a care provider. Unless health care professionals refer these patients for a comprehensive geriatric assessment and until clinicians consider the differential diagnosis of these presentations to include elder abuse, these "false negatives" will continue to occur. Unlike racism or gender issues, ageism is the single discrimination that all older persons will need to deal with.

In addition, over the past two decades, several studies have documented physicians' failure to diagnose a variety of common conditions in the elderly in the course of "usual and customary care." Examples include dementia, depression, and general functional decline. Geriatricians have conceptualized these entities as "geriatric syndromes," or common clinical problems that rarely have a single, underlying, pathophysiologic process, which is typically sought in the pure medical model. More often, there are several contributing factors that shape the clinical presentation. Typically, environmental factors play a prominent role. Interventions are multiple and directed at specific pathology, as well as contributing environmental factors.

Physicians and health care professionals may miss these common problems for several reasons. First, our professional training emphasizes the idea that a single diagnosis underlies all of the symptoms in any specific disease presentation, but this is rarely the case with the geriatric syndrome. Unlike many organic illnesses, their signs and symptoms may not be discussed in the course of the traditional office visit. Often these problems go unidentified or incompletely evaluated, because the older adult may offer few or many complaints, or may be brought in by family members that express vague concerns about general frailty or functional decline. Thus, elder abuse has many of the characteristics of a geriatric syndrome.

Framing elder abuse as a geriatric syndrome provides a conceptual starting point from which the physician and health care professional can begin to address mistreatment from screening to management. We must recognize that the definitive diagnosis and management requires a comprehensive evaluation of all potentially contributing factors. Again, the paradigm of the geriatric syndrome applies. The relative contribution of co-morbid medical conditions, environmental factors, and social influences must be determined before rational interventions are developed. Ideally a multi-disciplinary team, working effectively with adult protective service specialists, manages cases which present diagnostic challenges.

CLINICAL ASSESSMENT

As we frame *Elder Abuse* as a *geriatric syndrome*, let us turn our attention to the clinical assessment in the office setting. The same would hold true in other ambulatory settings across the continuum of care. As noted earlier, it is essential that we maintain a high index of suspicion for elder abuse, neglect, and financial exploitation. This holds true not only for the physician but for the professional staff as well. If we suspect elder abuse, recognize that the patient will be reluctant to reveal that abuse occurred and may retreat into a shell.

A quiet relaxing environment should be utilized. It is important to gain trust with the patient by using non-threatening questions. Clearly recognize that it is a red flag if a victim is not allowed to speak privately. After speaking with an elderly person about alleged abuse, never attempt to compare versions with the alleged abuser. In doing so, the alleged abuser will likely clue into the reason for your request. In turn, this may endanger the victim. In these discussions, it is critical to assume that the victim's statements are true and to make it clear that abuse is wrong and it is not the victim's fault. Victims need to be assured that they are not alone, and that help is available. In approaching a patient, it is essential to understand the underlying status of co-morbid medical and surgical conditions and review the patient's cognitive and functional status. If there is a decline, the trajectory of decline is essential to outline.

Undertake a thorough review of all medications, including over-the-counter medicines, herbs, and supplements and review the history of adherence to the medication regimen. In assessing for any history of alcohol and substance abuse, it is critical to understand the patient's perception of the problem. Many medications do not mix well with even small amounts of alcohol and can cause problems. It is important to be attentive to vague references to sexual advances or abuse and to elicit a history of any past history of neglect, abuse or domestic violence. As is the case of any geriatric syndrome, it is essential to get a complete psychosocial history. Since it is often related to elder abuse, it is important to assess for depression and anxiety as well as to recognize any longstanding relationship problems between the victim and perpetrator. The patient's perceived quality of life must be understood, as it may be clearly different than the health care professional's.

It is important to be aware of the level of caregiving required and the social support already in place. To fully understand the problem, it is also essential to appreciate the older persons' perception of the action and the cultural context in which the action occurred. In the assessment and management, it is critical to respect the patient, family and caregiver's spiritual and cultural beliefs. An inquiry about financial resources and the concerns that may stem from limitations in this regard should be obtained.

Finally and most importantly, mental capacity must be assessed. Mental capacity relates to a cluster of mental skills people use in everyday life, including memory, logic, ability to calculate, and the "flexibility" to turn attention from one task to another. Appropriate assessment of mental capacity is a complex process and not simply the mini-mental status exam. Because it is often difficult to determine, it is often a contentious issue. Strictly speaking, it is a medical determination and there is no standard "tool." Lack of capacity may lead one to live in squalor. From this clinician's perspective, honoring the wishes of person without capacity is a form of abandonment.

The physician must also assess the patient's ability to consent, as defined as someone accepts or agrees to something that somebody proposes. For legal and proper consent, the person consenting must have sufficient mental capacity and understand implications and ramifications of his/her actions. However, the older person may be under undue influence by an individual who is stronger or more powerful and prevails on the weaker individual to do something that the weaker person would not have done otherwise. This stronger individual may attempt techniques to isolate the weaker person, promote dependency or induce fear or distrust.

Undue influence and mental capacity are distinct. Both raise the question of whether the individual acted freely. While diminished capacity may contribute to a person's vulnerability to undue influence, cognitive assessment cannot identify undue influence. Only the courts decide undue influence.

In summary, capacity depends on ability to understand the act or transaction, the consequences of taking or not taking action, the consequences of making or not making the transaction, weigh choices and make a decision and commitment to the decision.

ASSESSMENT AND MANAGEMENT TOOL

An invitation to close the *First Annual Conference on Elder Abuse: The Role of the Health Care Professional* in April 2002, a national conference presented by the University of California, Irvine, provided an opportunity to develop and present tools that could be shared as part of a national toolkit for health care professionals. As a result of research for the national conference and the failure to find a tested, valid, reliable and easily generalizable instrument, a single page *Principles of Assessment and Management of Elder Abuse Tool* (see Tables 1 and 2) was developed that was "real world" and "user friendly." This tool was shared at the conference and made available to download on the MedAmerica website, *www.MedAmericaLTC.com*. More than

TABLE 1. Front Page of Elder Abuse "Tool"

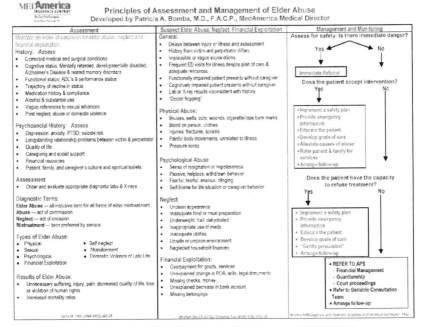

Copyright 2002 Patricia Bomba, M.D., F.A.C.P. / MedAmerica – All Rights Reserved – www.MedAmericaLTC.com

6000 laminated tools have been distributed to date, not including copies downloaded and reprinted with permission.

The assessment and management "tool" (Table 1 and 2) was developed for clinicians in busy practices and based on the author's experience in private practice in addition to community experience with clinical practice guidelines and principles. Development was based on a simple premise that a simple one-page "tool" that provides principles of assessment and management, best practice guidelines and screening questions will hopefully also serve to raise awareness of this important public health issue and maintain a high index of suspicion for elder abuse, neglect and financial exploitation. In our community, specialty advisory groups regularly review clinical practice guidelines for community-wide use and focus on the development of a single page tool accompanied by supporting materials. This approach has been well-received by busy practitioners. Better adherence to clinical practice guidelines has resulted.

TABLE 2. Back Page of Elder Abuse "Tool"

MEDAmerica Principles of Assessment and Management of Elder Abuse
Developed by Patricia A. Bomba, M.D., F.A.C.P., MedAmerica Medical Director

As health care professionals, our challenge is to balance:
1. Duty to protect to protect the safety of the vulnerable elder
2. Elder's right to self-determination

VALUES
- Treat elders with honesty, compassion, respect
- Goals of care should focus on improving quality of life and reducing suffering

PRINCIPLES: Rights of Older Adults
- Right to be safe
- Retain civil and constitutional rights, unless restricted by courts
- Can make decisions that do not conform to social norms if no harm to others
- Have decision-making capacity unless courts decide otherwise
- May accept or refuse services

BEST PRACTICE GUIDELINES
- First, DO NO HARM
- Interest of the senior is the priority
- Avoid imposing your personal values
- Respect diversity
- Involve the senior in the plan of care
- Establish short-term and long-term goals
- Recognize the senior's right to make choices
- Use family and informal support
- Recommend community-based services before institutional-based services, whenever possible
- In the absence of known wishes, act in the best interest and use substituted judgment

Adapted and modified from A National Association of Adult Protective Services Administrators (NAAPSA) consensus statement

SCREENING QUESTIONS:
- Are you afraid of anyone in your family?
- Has anyone close to you tried to hurt or harm you recently?
- Has anyone close to you called you names or put you down or made you feel bad recently?
- Does someone in your family make you stay in bed or tell you you're sick when you know you aren't?
- Has anyone forced you to do things you didn't want to do?
- Has anyone taken things that belong to you without your OK?

Modified 15-item H-S/EAST screening tool by Australian Women's Health Survey (Scofield, 1998)

Distribution of the tool has been accomplished through several distribution channels including a corporate distribution and fulfillment process, a corporate website, distribution of a physician elder abuse toolkit, awareness raised at regional, state and national conferences, and an electronic newsletter dedicated to promoting awareness of elder abuse and palliative care. In addition to physicians, nurses, social workers, Adult Protective Services workers, law enforcement and banking agencies, and community organizations hosting symposia on elder abuse have requested the tool. Subsequent to the presentation in California, additional opportunities to present nationally emerged. In addition to many parts of New York, requests for tools have come from many states and provinces including, but not limited to California, Arizona, Texas, Pennsylvania, Illinois, Florida, Maryland, Ohio, Delaware, Oregon, Missouri, Wyoming, North Carolina, Idaho, New Jersey, and Calgary, Alberta, Canada. The tool was translated into Russian and shared during educational training sessions held in Veiliky Novgorod, Russia as part of a sister city program between Rochester, New York and Veiliky Novgorod, Russia.

Feedback obtained indicated that the tool is useful not only for physicians but also for health care professionals working in both health care and long-term care systems. Community-based social workers, as well as emergency medical system, police, and banking personnel and others committed to combating this hidden epidemic have also found the tool helpful.

WHEN TO SUSPECT ELDER MISTREATMENT

Health care professionals in both systems and the community must recognize when to suspect elder abuse, neglect, and financial exploitation (Ejaz et al., 2001). Thus, examples of situations when elder mistreatment should be suspected were included on the tool.

In general, the presence of elder mistreatment must be considered whenever there are unreasonable delays in seeking medical attention between the injury or illness and the clinical assessment. Suspicion should be aroused when the history from the victim and the perpetrator significantly differs or there are implausible or vague explanations. If there are frequent emergency room visits for exacerbation of chronic disease despite a comprehensive plan for medical care and adequate resources, the clinician must be concerned about the possibility of elder mistreatment, particularly if different facilities are used. Take into account elder neglect when a functionally impaired or cognitively impaired patient presents for follow-up without a caregiver. Bear in mind the possibility when lab or X-ray results are inconsistent with the history and physical exam. Furthermore, when patients practice "doctor hopping" or frequent changes in clinicians, many factors should be considered including that it may be a result of confrontation of suspected elder mistreatment.

Bruises, welts, cuts, wounds, cigarette, and rope burn marks should easily raise suspicion, particularly if they are present at multiple sites, are bilateral, or shaped like objects (such as a belt or fingers). Injuries including fractures, strains, and dislocations, particularly those involving the upper body and untreated injuries in various stages of healing must signal concern to the health care professional. Painful body movements unrelated to illness and a change in demeanor or activity level should also raise suspicion.

Blood on the person or torn, stained, or bloody underclothing may be a manifestation of sexual abuse. Other manifestations might include:

- Bruises around the breasts, genitals, or inner thighs
- Unexplained venereal disease or genital infections
- Vaginal bleeding or unexplained anal bleeding
- Difficulty in walking or sitting without evidence of musculoskeletal disease.

Discussing sexual issues openly is difficult for many elderly women as they were raised in a time when the topic was taboo. Becoming a victim of sexual abuse represents not only the worse crime possible, but also the worst form of lost dignity and is unfathomable. Often there are feelings of profound shame or embarrassment that family, friends, or the community will discover the abuse and they will be shunned.

Psychological abuse results from verbal assaults, insults, threats, intimidation, humiliation, or harassment. It also results from intentionally isolating or ignoring an elder person, failing to provide companionship, making unannounced changes in routine, or failing to provide important information. One should suspect this type of abuse when a person exhibits a sense of resignation or hopelessness as well as passive, helpless, withdrawn behavior or appears fearful, tearful, anxious, or clinging. As a result, too often victims blame themselves for their life situation or caregiver behavior.

An unclean appearance resulting from poor personal hygiene may signify neglect. Inadequate food or meal preparation may result in underweight or malnourished, frail, dehydrated elders. In addition, pressure sores and general deterioration of health status result. Manifestations also include inappropriate or misuse of medications, unattended or untreated health problems or failure to provide necessary prosthetic devices, dentures, glasses, hearing aids, or durable medical equipment. Inadequate utilities (e.g., improper wiring, no heat, and no running water) lead to hazardous or unsafe living conditions. Unsafe or unclean environment (e.g., dirt, fleas, lice on the person, soiled bedding, fecal/urine smell, and inadequate clothing) can result in unsanitary living conditions and a public health hazard. Neglected household finances can add to the problem.

Seniors are vulnerable to overpayment for goods and services or provision of unnecessary services by scams and con artists. Financial exploitation must be considered if there is an abrupt or unexplained change in power of attorney, wills or other legal or financial documents. It must be suspected if there is discovery of an elder's signature forged for financial transactions or for titles to the elder's possessions. Missing checks or money, credit card bills from clothing or electronic equipment suppliers not likely to be frequented by the elder are all signs of financial abuse. An unexplained decrease in a bank account should raise a red flag. It may result from an unexplained withdrawal of large sums of money by a person accompanying the elder, by the unauthorized withdrawal of funds using an elder's ATM card, or by the unexplained sudden transfer of assets to a family member or someone outside the family. Missing belongings, particularly the unexplained disappearance of valuable possessions, must raise concern.

MANAGEMENT OF ELDER ABUSE

There are three essential questions to consider when one suspects elder mistreatment:

1. Is the patient safe?
2. Does the patient accept intervention?
3. Does the patient have the capacity to refuse treatment?

If there is immediate danger, there is need for immediate action and referral for appropriate intervention. If the patient is safe, there is time to develop trust and relationship with the patient and the caregiver. If the patient accepts intervention, the health care professional must implement a safety plan, provide emergency information, educate the patient that abuse is wrong, develop goals of care, alleviate the cause of abuse, refer the patient and family for appropriate services and importantly, arrange follow-up. If the patient refuses intervention and has capacity, the same series of steps exists along with "gentle persuasion" to accept intervention and importantly to arrange a follow-up appointment. A follow-up phone call from the physician, the physician extender or the nurse is often helpful in these situations. If the patient refuses intervention and lacks capacity, the clinician should refer the patient to Adult Protective Services, including arrangements for financial management, guardianship, and advocacy for possible court proceedings. In this situation, referral to a geriatric consultation team for comprehensive assessment may be helpful, if such consultation is available. Close follow-up of these high-risk cases is critical to a successful outcome.

PRINCIPLES AND BEST PRACTICE

As noted earlier, the challenge for health care professionals is to balance the duty to protect the safety of the vulnerable elder with the elder's right to self-determination. To do so effectively, health care professionals must commit to basic values, including treating elders with honesty, compassion, and respect and recognizing that goals of care should focus on improving quality of life and reducing suffering.

While recognizing the variations in disciplines, the National Association of Adult Protective Services Administrators (NAAPSA) consensus statement outlines basic principles and best practice guidelines that are meaningful for all health care practitioners and other professionals concerned with this growing public health issue. For that reason, a modified version was adapted for inclusion on the single page *Principles of Assessment and Management of Elder Abuse Tool.* The principles are based on the right of older adults and include:

- The right to be safe
- The right to retain civil and constitutional rights, unless restricted by the courts
- The right to make decisions that do not conform to social norms if no harm is brought to others
- The assumption that decision-making capacity is present, unless the courts decide otherwise and
- The older adult may accept or refuse services.

The best practice guidelines include:

- First, DO NO HARM
- The interest of the senior is the priority
- Avoid imposing your personal values
- Respect diversity
- Involve the senior in the plan of care
- Establish short-term and long-term goals of care
- Recognize the senior's right to make choices
- Use family and informal support
- Recommend community-based services before institutional-based services, whenever possible
- In the absence of known wishes, act in the best interest and use substituted judgment.

SCREENING QUESTIONS

Many different screening and assessment instruments have been developed to assist health care professionals in identifying elder abuse. The Hwalek-Sengstock Elder Abuse Screening Test (Hwalek & Sengstock, 1986) is a 15-item instrument to measure physical abuse, vulnerability and potential abusive situations. Further analysis and study yielded a 6-item brief, rapid screening instrument (Scofield et al., 1999). From a clinician's perspective, maintaining a high index of suspicion and consistently screening with a brief instrument that can be accomplished in a relatively short period of time is critical. For these reasons, these six screening questions were included:

1. Are you afraid of anyone in your family?
2. Has anyone close to you tried to hurt or harm you recently?
3. Has anyone close to you called you names or put you down or made you feel bad recently?
4. Does someone in your family make you stay in bed or tell you you're sick when you know you aren't?
5. Has anyone forced you to do things you didn't want to do?
6. Has anyone taken things that belong to you without your OK?

While a recent review of elder abuse screening and assessment instruments concludes that there is much to be done in terms of achieving consensus on what constitutes appropriate screenings (Fulmer et al., 2004), including routine screening questions does more than screen for elder mistreatment. Doing so provides a signal to the elder that it is a safe topic to explore with the health care professional, allowing other areas to be explored and a more detailed diagnostic assessment when necessary.

CONCLUSION

Health care professionals are in a unique position to identify and intervene on behalf of their patients. To do so, all health care professionals must maintain a high index of suspicion for elder abuse, neglect and financial exploitation in all settings across the continuum of care, including the community. To assure effective integration and coordination, all professionals must be prepared to work as part of an interdisciplinary team. Physicians, nurses, and social workers alike must recognize when to refer patients for additional assessment from colleagues and when and how to use community resources such as Adult Protective Services effectively. Equally important, health care professionals must be prepared to work with other professionals in the community, accepting appropriate referrals for more detailed diagnostic assessments. While signs of elder mistreatment are associated with a diminishing social network and poor social functioning, the older person's health status can be a contributing factor. Unrecognized and untreated depression, dementia, hypothyroidism in addition to polypharmacy and misuse of medications are examples of geriatric syndromes that are potential contributors and need medical input. The single page *Principles of Assessment and Management of Elder Abuse Tool* is a practical clinical tool that is available for use. It provides principles of assessment and management, best practice guidelines and screening questions that will hopefully serve to raise awareness of this important public health issue and help the practitioner maintain a high index of suspicion for elder abuse, neglect, and financial exploitation.

REFERENCES

Bureau of the Census (1997). Aging in the United States: Past, present, and future. Retrieved on May 8, 2005, from *www.census.gov/ipc/prod/97agewc.pdf*.

Center to Advance Palliative Care (2002). The case for hospital-based palliative care. Retrieved May 8, 2005, from *www.capc.org*.

Centers for Disease Control and Prevention (2005). Life expectancy hits record high. Retrieved May 8, 2005, from *http://www.cdc.gov/od/oc/media/pressrel/fs050228.htl*.

Education on Palliative and End-of-Life Care (EPEC) (n.d.). The EPEC project home page. Retrieved on May 8, 2005, from *http://epec.net/EPEC/webpages/index.cfm*.

Ejaz, F. K., Bass, D. M., Anetzberger, G. J., and Nagpaul, K. (2001). Evaluating the Ohio elder abuse and domestic violence in late life screening tool and referral protocol. *Journal of Elder Abuse & Neglect, 13*(2), 39-57.

Field, M. J., and Cassel, C. K. (Eds.) (1997). *Approaching death: Improving care at the end-of-life*. Washington, DC: National Academy Press.

Finger Lakes Health Systems Agency (2004). How will an aging population affect health care? Retrieved May 8, 2005, from *http://www.flhsa.org/pubs/aging*.

Fitch, K., Pyenson, B., Abbs, S., and Liang, M. (2004). Obesity: A big problem getting bigger. Milliman Research Report. Retrieved May 8, 2005, from *http://www.workforce.com/tools/obesityreport.pdf*.

Fulmer, T., Guadagno, L., Dyer, C., and Connolly, M. T. (2004). Progress in elder abuse screening and assessment instruments. *Journal of American Geriatrics Society, 52*, 297-304.

Hwalek, M., and Sengstok, M. (1986). Assessing the probability of abuse of the elderly: Towards the development of a clinical screening instrument. *Journal of Applied Gerontology 1986, 5*, 153-73.

Kaplan, L. O., and Peres, J. R. (2002). Means to a better end: A report on dying in America today. Washington, DC: Last Acts. Retrieved on May 8, 2005, from *http://www.rwjf.org/publications/otherlist.jsp*.

Lachs, M. S. (1995). Preaching to the unconverted: Educating physicians about elder abuse. *Journal of Elder Abuse & Neglect, 7*, 1-12.

Lachs, M. S. (1998). The mortality of elder abuse. *Journal of the American Medical Association, 280*(5), 428-32.

MedAmericaLTC. (n.d.). MedAmerica long-term care home page. Retrieved on May 8, 2005, from *http://www.yourlongtermcare.com/specialfeatures*.

National Center on Elder Abuse (n.d.). Retrieved May 8, 2005, from *www.elderabusecenter.org/basic/index.html*.

National Research Council (2003). *Elder mistreatment: Abuse, neglect, and exploitation in an aging America*. Panel to Review Risk and Prevalence of Elder Abuse and Neglect. Bonnie, R. J. and Wallace, R. B. (Eds.). Committee on National Statistics and Committee on Law and Justice, Division of Behavioral and Social Sciences and Education. Washington, DC: The National Academies Press.

Scofield, M., Reynolds, R., Michra, G. et al. (1999). Vulnerability to abuse, powerlessness, and psychological stress among older women. *Women's Health Australia Study*. Callagan, New South Wales, Australia: University of Australia.

Tartara, T., Thomas, C. et al. (1998). *National elder abuse incidence study: Final Report*. Washington, DC: National Center on Elder Abuse, American Public Human Services Association.

An Elder Abuse Shelter Program:
Build It and They Will Come,
A Long Term Care Based Program
to Address Elder Abuse in the Community

Daniel A. Reingold, MSW, JD

SUMMARY. This article describes how The Hebrew Home for the Aged at Riverdale (the Hebrew Home), a non-profit geriatric care center, has established one of the nation's first long term care based elder abuse prevention and intervention programs for elderly living in the community. This program, known as the Weinberg Center for Prevention, Intervention and Research in Elder Abuse (the "Weinberg Center"), received start-up funding in the form of a matching grant challenge from the Weinberg Foundation of Baltimore, which has a history of funding innovative geriatric programs throughout the United States. Utilizing the Hebrew Home's extensive integrated service model, a multidisciplinary team works with a network of private and governmental agencies. This model was designed based upon the needs of this population as described in the nascent research, evaluation of the few programs in existence, and the emerging state of elder abuse as a matter of public policy. The goals are to increase public awareness, intervene to make the home safe, and provide a secure and fulfilling short or long term shelter. Re-

[Haworth co-indexing entry note]: "An Elder Abuse Shelter Program: Build It and They Will Come, A Long Term Care Based Program to Address Elder Abuse in the Community." Reingold, Daniel A. Co-published simultaneously in *Journal of Gerontological Social Work* (The Haworth Press, Inc.) Vol. 46, No. 3/4, 2006, pp. 123-135 ; and: *Elder Abuse and Mistreatment: Policy, Practice, and Research* (ed: M. Joanna Mellor, and Patricia Brownell) The Haworth Press, Inc., 2006, pp. 123-135. Single or multiple copies of this article are available for a fee from The Haworth Document Delivery Service [1-800-HAWORTH, 9:00 a.m. - 5:00 p.m. (EST). E-mail address: docdelivery@haworthpress.com].

search in prevalence and efficacious use of the shelter is being conducted. *[Article copies available for a fee from The Haworth Document Delivery Service: 1-800-HAWORTH. E-mail address: <docdelivery@haworthpress.com> Website: <http://www.HaworthPress.com> © 2006 by The Haworth Press, Inc. All rights reserved.]*

KEYWORDS. Elder abuse, elder neglect, elder abuse shelter, multidisciplinary team, nursing homes, social service collaboration, legal rights, social workers' role in elder abuse prevention

INTRODUCTION

The hidden epidemic of elder abuse, although existing for many years, has begun to attract public attention only recently, and even so, on a limited scale. Despite headline-grabbing horror stories, the federal government only began to identify and categorize elder abuse with the adoption of the 1987 amendments to the Older American Act. The establishment of an Elder Abuse Task Force in 1990 by the federal Department of Health and Human Services, and the creation of the National Institute on Elder Abuse in 1991 legislatively identified elder abuse as a critical dilemma requiring an immediate policy response (Daniels, 1999).

With governmental attention, and recognition of the compelling demographics, literature emerged with empirical and anecdotal studies. Increasing awareness of this national epidemic spawned theories and research addressing risk factors and abuser profiles (National Academy of Science, 2003). In addition, with great creativity and ingenuity (and grossly inadequate funding) small community-based social work, legal and medical programs began to address the social crisis (Teaster, 2003). Devotion of the *Journal of Gerontological Social Work* to the issue of elder abuse is a testament to the growing contribution of the social work profession to the intellectual and programmatic discourse.

Despite all of these important contributions, elder abuse is, today, where child abuse and domestic violence were 25 years ago: there are only a limited number of states with mandatory reporting of community-based elder abuse (Teaster, 2003), there is no definitive conclusion on prevalence (Brownell, 2004), there is ambiguity as to definition (Loue, 2001), and there is debate as to what constitutes the most effective intervention (Brownell, 2004). Unlike the genesis of programs for child abuse, a review of the literature reveals few if any elder abuse shelters in the United States. Furthermore the long term care setting is underutilized as an intervention in community-based elder abuse. Throughout all of North America, only one–the Kirby Center in Calgary, Alberta–appears in the literature as a shelter currently operated by a larger agency for seniors. Kirby's data shows that for elder abuse, a multi-disciplinary model is the most effective intervention.

If the child and spouse abuse programs are any indication, the success of elder abuse intervention is encouraging. The successes, thus far, of reducing the incidents of child and spouse abuse since 1975 (although the number of reports is growing) can be ascribed to a dramatic increase in public awareness and education as well as training of multi-disciplined professionals (Wolf, 1996).

The challenges, then, among many in this underserved arena, are to increase public education and awareness, determine how to find victims, gain trust and access, encourage them to accept service, and develop a safe emergency shelter. These are the goals of the Weinberg Center.

DISCUSSION

Historical Overview of The Hebrew Home's Elder Abuse Initiatives

The Hebrew Home's establishment of the Weinberg Center is a culmination of the Home's historic roots in addressing the needs of neglected elderly. The Hebrew Home was established in 1917 in Harlem as a shelter for homeless and neglected Jewish elderly. In 1950, the Hebrew Home relocated to a 20 acre campus in the Riverdale section of the Bronx. Today, the Hebrew Home provides a full continuum of residential healthcare, home care and housing options on a non-profit, non-sectarian basis. Together with its ElderServe community services division, the Hebrew Home serves over 3,000 older people throughout Manhattan, the Bronx, and Westchester County.

In 1996, recognizing the need to focus multi-disciplinary professional and governmental attention on elder abuse, the Hebrew Home sponsored a day long conference in New York City. A panel of professionals was assembled to discuss this insidious and rapidly growing problem. It became evident that much work was needed to define, identify and report elder abuse, and to conduct training in those areas.

In the following year, the Hebrew Home partnered with the Westchester County District Attorney's Office to create a pilot project to educate law enforcement professionals about elder abuse. Westchester County was selected because its demographic profile–20 percent of its residents are elderly–is a precursor to our nation's demographics in 2015 when the front end of the baby boomers reach age 70. The award-winning program has continued for the past seven years to educate the public, law enforcement, and health care professionals about the signs and symptoms of various forms of abuse.

In 1999, the Bronx District Attorney's Office, seeing a sharp increase in crimes against the elderly in that borough, requested the Hebrew Home's assistance in replicating the Westchester program and it has since been an integral part of that prosecutor's office. Educational seminars are scheduled throughout the year and printed materials defining elder abuse and providing emergency referral information are distributed to law enforcement personnel.

Prior to the inception of the Hebrew Home's elder abuse prevention program, there was a dearth of discrete legal material to be used in prosecuting elder abuse cases, a minimal relationship between the legal and medical/social service professions, and a lack of a unified vocabulary. In addition, prosecution of elder abuse cases is in the best of circumstances complex as it often involves victims with dementia and reliance on circumstantial evidence. Since then, the seminars presented by the Hebrew Home in conjunction with the Westchester and Bronx District Attorneys' offices, together with the greater education and awareness of law enforcement professionals around the country, have resulted in the development of better legal resources which have been used successfully to prosecute cases (Stiegal, 2000).

The Hebrew Home partnered with a member of the New York State Legislature in 2000 to implement the "Watchful Eye" program, in which peepholes were installed in hundreds of inner-city apartments to prevent so-called "push-in" crimes against the elderly. During the installation of these peepholes, Hebrew Home professionals met with homebound elders to teach safety precautions, and to perform home assessments. Based on that experience, a large-print safety checklist for homebound elderly was developed and distributed throughout our service area.

In 2001, the Hebrew Home secured support from an area bank and conducted training sessions for bank tellers to recognize financial abuse. This program helped sensitize bank tellers to improper bank withdrawals–including, for example, a client, suffering from dementia, who "approved" of a fraudulent third-party withdrawal.

Establishment of The Weinberg Center

In 2004, the Hebrew Home recognized the need to formalize its commitment to intervening in elder abuse cases, and understood that in addition to effective training, we had the capability, through our comprehensive delivery system, to provide direct intervention in cases of abuse and neglect. Moreover, our success in building strong collaborative relationships with other specialized non-profit agencies and with our governmental colleagues, established a strong foundation on which to build a comprehensive elder abuse program. The completion of a series of new building projects on the Hebrew Home campus enabled us to establish one of the nation's first long term care based shelters for victims.

Building on the organization's existing geriatric services, the Hebrew Home developed an array of new programs: emergency protective shelter services; an integrated continuum of care for victims of elder abuse and neglect; unique elder abuse detection, prevention, and intervention strategies; expanded training initiatives for law enforcement and community-based individuals; and, research to profile victims and assess the efficacy of these programs.

Adoption of Multidisciplinary Team Approach

The use of multidisciplinary teams "has become a hallmark of elder abuse prevention programs, reflecting growing consensus that no single agency or discipline has all the resources or expertise needed to effectively resolve all forms of abuse and neglect" (Nerenberg, p. 3, 2003). It is suggested that such teams may be in a better position to accurately assess elder abuse (Fulmer, 1999).

With that knowledge, the initial decision of the Weinberg Center was to adopt a multidisciplinary team approach. From the social work/therapeutic perspective, this was a decision with at least three benefits: accuracy of assessment; efficient staff allocation; and, an inherent support mechanism.

> When people of different backgrounds and expertise get together, they learn from each other's expertise. It can increase the range of options in dealing with these very complicated [abuse] cases. Teams that meet regularly develop relationships with one another that ultimately benefit the client.
>
> Working in a team can offer emotional relief when professionals feel angry, helpless, or frustrated with the client. (Dick-Muehlke, p. 129, 1996)

The multidisciplinary team at the Weinberg Center is comprised of the following: Nurse Administrator, Social Worker, Adult Day Care Director (Nurse), Geriatrician Attorney (Liaison with Pace Women's Justice Center), Community Service Liaison (Nurse), Intake/Admissions (Nurse).

The Weinberg Center currently collaborates with the following agencies:

Bronx District Attorney

Manhattan District Attorney

New York City Adult Protective Services

New York Well Cornell Medical Center, Division of Geriatrics and Gerontology

Pace Women's Justice Center

Westchester Adult Protective Services

Westchester District Attorney

Westchester County Department of Senior Programs and Services

This group is continually growing. For example, we are developing a relationship with the community hospital division of a large academic medical center which is in our 911 catchment area. Our goal there is to create an area of elder abuse expertise within the emergency room and among the hospitals. Any agency which has specialized services and is interested in helping is welcome at the table.

Access to the Weinberg Center

Fundamental to the success of the Weinberg Center is its capability to make information and services for victims of elder abuse easily accessible. The Hebrew Home has secured a recognizable toll-free number *(1-800-56-SENIOR)*. The phone number has been disseminated to area Adult Protective Services (APS) because APS has recognition in the field and legal authority which enables them to be the first responder. Once APS determines that intervention from the Weinberg Center is needed, they will contact, or refer the caller to the Center. In addition, the phone number was distributed to emergency rooms, and local domestic violence and elder advocacy agencies. Telephone service is staffed 24/7 for immediate response to all inquiries. This is the initial contact point for crisis intervention and provides the caller prompt access to the Weinberg Center or other appropriate referral. It also enables the Weinberg Center to conduct screening to determine if elder abuse services are indicated, or if less emergent intervention can be offered. The telephone mechanism also provides a centralized opportunity to collect data which will be analyzed and evaluated by the Home's Research Division.

Once contact has been made with the Weinberg Center, either by or on behalf of a victim of abuse or neglect, and a determination made that emergency shelter is needed, triage is performed in the Hebrew Home's ElderServe medical day program. Operating 24/7, the ElderServe medical day program is staffed by registered nurses, a social worker and a full array of healthcare professionals who have been specially trained to address the emergent needs of victims in the first 24-48 hours. Comfortable, secure and attractive overnight suites for men and women were constructed. A multidisciplinary assessment of the victim is performed to assure their health status and arrange for placement in the short term stay unit (described below), or, if appropriate, for their return home with support from ElderServe's other community-based programs. In some cases, victims already have been assessed by medical personnel, again, utilizing the multidisciplinary approach to care and resource allocation.

Legal Advocacy

Within the multidisciplinary design of the Weinberg Center, The Pace Women's Justice Center (PWJC) provides civil legal support. PWJC brought considerable expertise, as it has a long history of providing comprehensive legal services for victims of domestic violence and other forms of abuse. A PWJC attorney who has extensive experience as a former elder abuse prosecutor in the Manhattan District Attorneys' office, was assigned to the Weinberg Center. PWJC can provide or arrange for legal assistance for victims referred to the Weinberg Center including obtaining orders of protection, securing temporary financial maintenance, and seeking other necessary legal remedies.

This collaborative relationship with PWJC has contributed significantly to the successful impact of the Weinberg Center program. In addition to offering civil legal expertise, the participation of PWJC gives access to their panel of elder law attorneys, who can provide legal service beyond the capability of the Weinberg Center, and who have referred cases of abuse or neglect where caregiving was needed.

Short Term Stay

The Center's short term stay unit offers safe and secure emergency housing, respite and support for seniors who are experiencing abuse or neglect in their homes. Short term stays are for approximately thirty days. The Center is located on the main campus of the Hebrew Home, which is gated and secure.

Lengthy consideration was made as to where to house the victims within the Hebrew Home campus. An existing 31-bed wing of the Hebrew Home was initially adapted for use as an elder abuse shelter. In actuality, fewer beds were necessary on the dedicated unit, and other short term care residents are housed there as well.

Ultimately, it appears integration with other residents best serves the needs of the abused population. This integration had two benefits. First, the needs of clients referred to the Weinberg Center are diverse. While some clients are cognitively and physically intact, many who have been self-neglecting are frail, and require extensive assistance with activities of daily living, nutrition, physical rehabilitation, as well as legal and psychological services. Others pre- sent with various stages of dementia. While the short term stay unit is staffed, equipped and designed for the former group, clients suffering with dementia are referred to one of the Hebrew Home special care units, which are more responsive to their needs. Again, the use of the multidisciplinary team assures a better assessment and referral. Their ongoing case-management and interface with the Hebrew Home direct care staff assures that the additional elder abuse- related services, such as legal, psychological, and/or financial, are part of the client's care plan. The second benefit is integration of clients–many of whom have been isolated–into the social fabric of the Hebrew Home community. Thus stigma is avoided, and social support is fostered.

Clients are fully integrated with other residents living in the Hebrew Home, and enjoy the same gracious lifestyle and clinical services. They have a complete medical assessment and are invited to participate in all recreational programs and special events. A plan of care, including transfer to other residential options (described below) if appropriate, is developed with each client. The plan of care may include support groups, counseling, or civil legal services. The goal is to ensure their sense of personal freedom, safety and full use of the Home's facilities as a sanctuary from their previous environments, where they were likely to have felt physically or mentally at-risk, isolated, and dependent.

Long Term Care Plan

The multidisciplinary team develops a plan of care for each guest during their short term stay. At the completion of the thirty days (or such shorter or longer stay, as is indicated), the plan of care delineates one of three possible next steps:

(A) return to the clients' home, if safe, with community support services and oversight offered by ElderServe;
(B) transfer to one of four specially designated apartments in RiverWalk, the Hebrew Home's senior housing community; or,
(C) long-term admission to the Hebrew Home's residential healthcare facility.

Returning Home with Community Support Services

Either after triage at the time of initial referral, or following short term stay, clients for whom return to their own home is appropriate and safe are referred to ElderServe, the Hebrew Home's community services division. Under the coordination of the ElderServe care manager, ElderServe offers a full range of services for victims in their own homes including access to one of Elder-Serve's conveniently located community sites and additional counseling and legal advocacy. This referral is particularly effective where the client has suffered from self-neglect (whether due to physical frailty or dementia) or where the abuser has been removed from an otherwise safe housing situation. The ElderServe home health care programs offer a full range of health care, social and supportive services, medical management, nursing services, rehabilitation therapies, and personal care in a client's own home. The home care team assists with the personal activities of daily living and offers a comprehensive range of healthcare and personal care services.

ElderServe's five medical and social model adult day programs provide meals, transportation, social and recreational programs for clients who might otherwise be socially isolated. Adult day programs are available 24/7, and round trip, door-to-door transportation is provided.

Transfer to RiverWalk

Located on the Hebrew Home's main campus, RiverWalk is a 137-unit senior housing community. For clients who cannot safely return home, but who do not need long term residential healthcare, referrals are made to an apartment in RiverWalk for temporary or permanent housing.

Four one-bedroom apartments were renovated and reserved for this purpose. Clients referred to RiverWalk have a safe and attractive apartment that includes congregate meals, area transportation, housekeeping, social work, and recreation services.

Admission to Hebrew Home

Clients who are not able to return home safely, or who need additional support services not available in RiverWalk, are given priority access to the Hebrew Home's long term residential health care services. Placement in the Hebrew Home ensures a comprehensive and coordinated system of 24-hour nursing care, which includes physician services, and access to the Home's activities and events. Supplemental counseling, including legal advocacy for elder abuse victims, is provided.

Rationale for the Long Term Care Venue

Creation of the Weinberg Center within the rubric of a large, fully integrated long-term care setting is an exciting model that should be replicated in other communities. The expense of building and operating a stand-alone shelter is prohibitive. Zoning issues, access to construction capital, developing an operating income stream and staffing on a 24/7 basis are formidable challenges.

Every community has a ready supply of existing nursing homes, many with additional home care and housing services. Nursing homes bring to the elder abuse equation specialized understanding of the needs of physically frail, an ongoing 24/7 operation, and environments which are specially designed for frail elderly, those with dementia, and even those who only need minimal support. Equally important, nursing homes have developed expertise in addressing elder abuse, having been directed by legislation and regulation, to engage in mandatory reporting and investigation for almost twenty years.

The notion of the nursing home as a safe-haven for victims of elder abuse or neglect should be embraced for today's elder abuse crisis. Unless other forms of funding become available for construction and operation of shelters, nursing homes offer an immediate, attractive, and suitable solution for all elder abuse victims. In particular, non-profit long term care facilities such as the Hebrew Home offer a wide array of services which can be adapted, as with the Weinberg Center, to offer efficient intervention. Provision of this type of service furthers the eleemosynary mission and purpose of non-profit homes, and supports our tax exempt status. Many non-profit homes have embraced the "Quality First" initiative launched by the American Association of Homes and Services for the Aging, the national trade association for non-profit homes. "Quality First" is a covenant in which a commitment is made to the community and other stakeholders to provide the finest and most efficient care possible. Programs to combat elder abuse and alleviate community-based self-neglect completely support Quality First.

Programs and services in nursing homes have advanced dramatically over the past ten years, particularly in the non-profit world. Initiatives such as the Eden Alternative, Pioneers, and EverCare, have created environments which are resident-centered, customer service oriented and positive (Kane, 1998). Professionals in the field of elder abuse have "observed that often nursing home placement resulted in dramatic improvement in quality of life that was apparent to all observers . . ." (Lachs, 2002).

In the Weinberg Center approach, long term care placement is the last option to be considered, after home care or housing has been ruled out as not in the best interest of the client.

Education and Support Program for Informal Caregivers

Elder abuse may stem from situations where there is lack of caregiving experience, knowledge, resources, or some other inability to provide an appropriate level of care. Research findings also support the notion that stressed or overburdened caregivers are more likely to abuse their relative, particularly when the underlying relationship is poor (Anetzberger, 2000). *Intent* to mistreat is not necessarily present. In such cases, intervention with the abuse victim and the "abuser" is critical, and can prove fruitful in securing the well-being of the caregiving dyad.

Operating within the "strengthening family ties" model, a training and education program is being developed as part of the Weinberg Center geared to the family or other informal caregiver. It will consist of training for informal caregivers to prevent the abusive situation, including caregiving training modules; support groups; individual counseling; stress-management; and, education about and referral to home care, respite or day care to alleviate pressure.

Public Education, Outreach, and Training

Mobile Outreach Van

In the field of elder abuse, it is a corollary that the most difficult group to reach are those who are most at-risk. Because of their isolation and/or dependence on the caregiver, the subjects most in need of help are the least accessible.

The Weinberg Center launched an outreach van, staffed by a trained nurse, social worker, and law student, which visits area senior centers, naturally occurring retirement communities, and malls to disseminate information about the Weinberg Center and to encourage referrals of shut-ins who may be abused, neglected, or at-risk. In addition, staff provides information and education and also can intervene immediately, if directed to an at-risk individual.

Community-Based Training

A key element of preventing and intervening in elder abuse cases is identification. As community-based abuse or neglect almost always occurs behind closed doors, access to that venue is key. Proper training of those who are in a unique position to observe and identify elder abuse and neglect is a critical element of public awareness, prevention, and intervention.

Local 32 B/J/E are the union locals that represent doormen, building superintendents and porters in residential buildings throughout Westchester County, the Bronx, and Manhattan. They are in a unique position to know what is taking place behind the closed doors of the apartment house. The Weinberg Center provides training for union members. Training gives hundreds of members the ability to define, identify and report cases of abuse or neglect. A public information campaign distributes printed material at all participating residential sites describing what to look for, and telephone numbers for reporting and referral. Cards have been produced for Local 32 members for their use and to share with letter carriers who work on routes with smaller buildings, which do not have doormen, superintendents, or porters.

Meals on Wheels Programs

Delivery of Meals on Wheels is an effective vehicle to identify abuse or neglect. Cards with information on abuse and neglect, and reporting information, are distributed to Meals on Wheels delivery personnel throughout the Bronx, Manhattan, and Westchester County.

Other Community-Based Training

The Weinberg Center's multidisciplinary team continues to develop nontraditional sources for training. Currently in discussion are training of pharmacists, hairdressers, dog-walking services, telephone technicians, and cable or utility installers.

Law Enforcement Training

As described, the Hebrew Home has partnered with the district attorney offices to conduct law enforcement training. These programs have educated the public, law enforcement, and health care professionals about the prevalence, and the signs and symptoms of various forms of abuse. The Weinberg Center has expanded this training to other governmental agencies and they, in turn, have provided training to our staff and constituency.

CONCLUSION

The Weinberg Center of the Hebrew Home has developed a proactive, vertically and horizontally integrated system of intervention, prevention and response for victims of elder abuse and neglect. This program will result in effective strategies to diminish the incidence of elder abuse and encourage replication at the regional and national levels. This program emphasizes a spectrum of programmatic and human resources, community affiliations and organizational endorsements which have resulted in a system of coordinated crisis intervention, residential and community based services, training, and community awareness that will ensure the provision of the right care, at the right time and in the right place for the victims of elder abuse and neglect. As with many other programs and services in the elder abuse arena, the Weinberg Center is in the early stage of its development. We welcome responses to our initiative: suggestions, sharing of other experiences, and critiques. We recognize that there are no right answers, only best practices. By working together, social work professionals, gerontologists, service providers, and the law enforcement community (both public and private) can make significant progress in reducing elder abuse and caring for its victims.

REFERENCES

Anetzberger, G.J. (2000). Caregiving: Primary cause of elder abuse? *Generations.*

Brownell, P., Welty, A., & Brennan, M. (2000). *Aging in New York State and Implications for Elder Abuse and Neglect.* New York State Office for the Aging, Project 2015.

Daniels, R.S., Baumhover, L.A., Formby, W.A., & Clark-Daniels, C.L. (1999). Police discretion and elder mistreatment. *Journal of Criminal Justice* Vol. 27. No. 3.

Dick-Muehlke, C., Yang, J. A., Yu, D., & Paul, D. (1996). Abuse of cognitively impaired elders: Recognition and intervention. *Silent Suffering: Elder Abuse in America,* Archstone Foundation.

Fulmer, T., Ramirez, M., Fairchild, S., Holmes, D., Koren, M.J., & Teresi, J. (1999). Prevalence of elder mistreatment as reported by social workers in a probability sample of adult day health care clients. *Journal of Elder Abuse & Neglect,* Vol. 11.

Kane, R., Kane, R., & Ladd, R. (1998). *The Heart of Long Term Care.* Oxford University Press.

Lachs, M.S., Williams, C. S., O'Brien, S., & Pillemer, K. (2002). Adult protective service use and nursing home placement. *The Gerontologist.*

Loue, S. (2001). Elder abuse and neglect in medicine and law. *Journal of Legal Medicine,* Vol. 22, pp. 159-209.

National Academy of Sciences. (2003). Executive summary. *Elder Mistreatment, Abuse, Neglect, and Exploitation in Aging in America.*

Nerenberg, L. (2003). Multidisciplinary elder abuse prevention teams–A new generation. *National Committee for the Prevention of Elder Abuse.*

Stiegal, L. (2000). The changing role of the courts in elder-abuse cases. *Generations.*

Teaster, P. B. (2003). *A Response to the Abuse of Vulnerable Adults: The 2000 Survey of State Adult Protective Services.* National Center on Elder Abuse.

Teaster, P. B., & Nerenberg, L. (2003). A national look at elder abuse multidisciplinary teams. *Report for the National Committee for the Prevention of Elder Abuse.*

Wolf, R. S. (1996). Strategies to prevent elder abuse in the community. *Silent Suffering: Elder Abuse in America.* Archstone Foundation.

Consumer Fraud and the Elderly:
A Review of Canadian Challenges
and Initiatives

Carole A. Cohen, MD

SUMMARY. Financial abuse is the most common type of elder abuse. Consumer fraud, a form of financial abuse perpetrated by criminals who do not know the victim, is not well studied. Seniors represent a disproportionate percentage of the victims of consumer fraud. This article reviews the data on the prevalence of consumer fraud (primarily telemarketing scams) in Canada. It examines the reasons why Canadian seniors are targets of fraud. It also describes many unique initiatives developed at the local, provincial and national level in Canada to educate seniors and those who care for them about the types of scams and the risks of fraud. *[Article copies available for a fee from The Haworth Document Delivery Service: 1-800-HAWORTH. E-mail address: <docdelivery@haworthpress.com> Website: <http://www.HaworthPress.com> © 2006 by The Haworth Press, Inc. All rights reserved.]*

KEYWORDS. Consumer fraud, elderly, Canada

[Haworth co-indexing entry note]: "Consumer Fraud and the Elderly: A Review of Canadian Challenges and Initiatives." Cohen, Carole A. Co-published simultaneously in *Journal of Gerontological Social Work* (The Haworth Press, Inc.) Vol. 46, No. 3/4, 2006, pp. 137-144 ; and: *Elder Abuse and Mistreatment: Policy, Practice, and Research* (ed: M. Joanna Mellor, and Patricia Brownell) The Haworth Press, Inc., 2006, pp. 137-144. Single or multiple copies of this article are available for a fee from The Haworth Document Delivery Service [1-800-HAWORTH, 9:00 a.m. - 5:00 p.m. (EST). E-mail address: docdelivery@haworthpress.com].

INTRODUCTION

Financial or material abuse of the elderly is recognized as the most common type of elder abuse (McDonald et al., 1991). Financial abuse can be perpetrated by someone who knows the victim and encompasses such acts as theft, misuse of power of attorney, forgery, extortion, and breach of trust. Someone who does not know the victim can also perpetrate financial abuse and exploitation of the elderly. This is classified as consumer fraud and is becoming recognized as a growing problem and concern. Consumer fraud encompasses telemarketing schemes such as lottery and prize scams, fake investment schemes involving property and stock, home renovation fraud, internet fraud, bank inspector schemes, public utility impostor scam, and many other schemes (National Advisory Council on Aging, 2001). Canada has been identified as home to many of these schemes. In fact, some argue that Toronto is the capital of consumer fraud (Mascoll, 1999). This article will review the extent of the problem in Canada and outline a number of initiatives that have been developed to educate seniors and others of the risks of these schemes.

EXTENT OF THE PROBLEM

Little is known about the extent of material abuse or victimization of seniors and this has been identified as deserving of study (Vida, 1994). Otiniano et al. (1998) surveyed 200 seniors attending Senior's Centres in Houston, Texas. From the 157 usable surveys 27% reported being victims of fraud in the past year. Ethnicity was significantly different among those who had been abused, with Hispanics being victims more often than African-Americans, Whites or Asians. The most common type of financial abuse was notification of fake prizes (20% of cases).

Podnieks et al. (1992) completed a telephone survey of 2000 older adults living in private dwellings in Canada. They found that 4% had experienced abuse and/or neglect since they turned sixty-five years of age. Material abuse was the most common abuse cited (2.5%). Six percent reported theft by strangers. The Canadian National Advisory Council on Aging Bulletin published an issue on fraud in 2001 (National Advisory Council on Aging). It reported that more than 50% of reported victims of fraudulent telemarketing were over sixty years of age and people over sixty accounted for three-quarters of those defrauded more than $5,000. The victims of home repair scams were usually women with an average age of 74.5 years and ninety-five percent lived alone. The victims of investment and securities fraud were noted to be male.

PhoneBusters (see below) has been collecting data on phone fraud in Canada for over five years. They report that since 1995 Canadians have lost about $40 million as a result of this type of fraud. In 2001, the last year that complete data is available, there were 194 cases of telemarketing fraud reported with a total dollar loss of $1,040,428 (Canadian dollars) (*www.phonebusters.com*). Ninety percent of the victims were over 60 years of age. Much less is known about victims of other types of fraud including renovation fraud, fake investments schemes and other types of fraud that have been described.

WHY ARE SENIORS TARGETS OF FRAUD IN CANADA?

Risk factors for elder abuse have been widely studied and researchers have identified psychiatric illness in the caregiver, issues related to caregiving situation or previous relationship, and social isolation of the caregiver as important. Victim characteristics include poor mental and physical health and problems between victim and the abuser (Vida, 1994). However, financial abuse is seen as very different than other forms of abuse in that social isolation of the victim is particularly important and the abuser is often not intimately associated with the victim. In these situations, caregiver burden is clearly not a factor.

Much less is known about elderly victims of consumer fraud. Offenders of telemarketing scams have told the police that the ideal target is an elderly person, living alone with limited contact with their family. Victims are also a high-risk group and victim information is often sold to other criminals (*www. phonebusters.com*). In one study of consumer fraud among patients of a community psychogeriatric service in Toronto, Ontario, there was a striking pattern among victims. They were all women with an average age of eighty- five, socially isolated with mild cognitive impairment. They all had designated power of attorney to someone but this person did not know of the abuse or of the need to provide increased supervision of financial affairs (Cohen, 2002).

Many other factors have been postulated to explain why seniors are ideal victims of consumer fraud (National Advisory Council on Aging, 2001). Women of this generation may not be as familiar with money management and used to turning such matters over to men whenever possible. They may be more reluctant to seek advice on financial matters. This generation also has significant financial resources and is very trusting of others. Their experiences during the Great Depression make them particularly vulnerable, as this was a time when one assisted strangers in need. Seniors are also very generous in their donations to legitimate charities. They may not be aware of consumer fraud as a crime so they do not recognize when they have been victims and fail to report it to the police. They may also fail to seek help because of embarrassment.

Although not specific to this type of abuse, identification of victims may be hampered by a number of additional factors related to the health and social systems. The Canadian prevention guidelines designed to assist Canadian physicians in their periodic health exam do not recommend screening for elder abuse (Canadian Task Force). They recommend instead that physicians be alert to the indications of abuse and take measures to prevent further abuse. However, one study of Canadian nonspecialist physicians in Hamilton, Ontario, identified many knowledge deficits related to elder abuse (Krueger et al., 1997). In this study, 52% of the respondents reported they had seen patients they suspected were victims of abuse. The family physicians reported several problems including not knowing where to get help if they suspected abuse, lack of protocols for dealing with abuse and the victims' denial of abuse and resistance to intervention. Only 45% said they were fairly or very confident in assessing whether elder abuse existed in their practice and only 22% were fairly or very confident about knowledge of existing community resources.

The justice system in Canada has also been identified as a factor in failing to protect seniors from elder abuse and consumer fraud. Laws that protect vulnerable seniors and legislate how those who are financially incompetent will be helped vary from province to province across Canada. This often causes confusion for those trying to assist vulnerable seniors. Consumer fraud is difficult to prosecute and Canada has a relatively low rate of prosecuting these criminals (National Advisory Council on Aging, 2001). For instance, there is a need to prosecute the telemarketing criminals in the jurisdiction where the telephone call was made and in Canada, this may be in another province at a great distance from the victim. Police forces may not be able to travel large distances to interview victims and victims often cannot travel to testify. Current banking regulations may also hinder investigations, as bank tellers who notice criminal transactions may not be able to report them because of privacy regulations.

The Toronto Star, a newspaper in Canada's largest city, has done some investigative work on the subject of telemarketing fraud (Mascoll, 1999). They quoted a United States postal inspector who told the court during a trial ". . . Toronto is becoming the world capital for telefraud with 50% of it perpetrated in United States cities." In one case, twenty-nine Toronto conmen bilked 84 female Americans out of a total of $1 million in life savings. Another story reported the plight of a postal carrier in Kingston, Ontario, who was suspended after she refused to deliver "scratch-and-win" cards (Bailey, 1999). These cards tell most recipients they are winners and urge them to call a 900-number to collect their prize. They do not inform the recipient of the potentially high cost of placing such a call. This is defined as a legal "grey area" as it is legal to mail these items in Canada. In a follow-up article in 2002 the *Toronto Star* still expressed concerns regarding lax sentencing of criminals who perpetuate telemarketing fraud (Cribb, 2002).

CANADIAN INITIATIVES TO PREVENT CONSUMER FRAUD

Medical and social interventions have been suggested to decrease the vulnerability of those at risk for elder abuse (Vida, 1994). These interventions would include informal supervision of an at risk senior, support to reduce their susceptibility to undue influence, education regarding their rights and actions they can take to protect themselves, removal from dangerous situations, protection via guardianship or other means if the competency of the senior is in question and application of the Criminal code to the extent possible.

Canada has developed some unique programs to combat deceptive telemarketing and educate seniors. PhoneBusters was founded by the Ontario Provincial Police in 1993 and is a national deceptive telemarketing call centre. Its original mandate was to prosecute criminals in the provinces of Ontario and Quebec involved in phone fraud using the Criminal Code of Canada. The mandate now includes facilitating prosecution of criminals by the United States (*www.phonebusters.com*). PhoneBusters is operated by volunteers and members of the Ontario Provincial Police. Members of the public can call Phone-Busters for information on phone fraud or to report a complaint. PhoneBusters collects data on telemarketing fraud in Canada and shares the information with the appropriate enforcement agency. Senior volunteers from SeniorBusters work with PhoneBusters to provide telephone support and information to victims of telemarketing fraud. Between October 1997 and May 2001, Senior-Busters reached 980 victims in the United States and 2101 victims in Canada (*www.phonebusters.com*).

The Competition Bureau of Canada is responsible for the Competition Act, which is the federal law that makes telemarketing fraud a crime. In 1996, the Competition Bureau and other agencies formed the Deceptive Telemarketing Prevention Forum. The Forum is made up of business, government and not-for-profit organizations. One of its goals is to educate the general public how to spot phone scams, what to do and how to report them. A social marketing campaign was launched by the Forum in 1998 with the release of a poster and pamphlet. A video entitled *Phone Fraud: It's a Trap* was launched more recently (*http://competition.ic.gc.ca*). The Forum sponsors education sessions, puts notices in bank statements and credit card bills and keeps statistics on telemarketing fraud. The Competition Bureau's Information Centre assists

PhoneBusters and the telephone numbers, web site and e-mail address of both organizations appears on all educational materials.

The Canadian Association of Retired Persons (CARP) held a national forum on scams and fraud in 1998. More than a hundred organizations from across Canada attended (MacAulay, 1998). The mission of the forum was to "develop practical and effective strategies in the fight against those who prey on vulnerable adults." Participants suggested strengthening treaties between Canada and the United States concerning cross-border fraudulent activities, education and information-sharing and networking between organizations represented at the forum to continue sharing information about fraud prevention. Call Block services are available to prevent calls being made to 1-900 or 1-976 numbers and are available for a minimal fee. CARP has asked Bell Canada to add a message to 976 to allow callers to hang up and to permit callers to 1-900 to be allowed more time to evaluate the message before they must hang up or be charged.

In 1999, an additional law, Bill C-20, was passed in Canada. It addressed some of the frequently raised concerns about the Canadian justice system. It has criminal provisions specifically dealing with telemarketing fraud. It provides for stiffer fines and jail terms and powers to investigate and shut down suspicious operators. It allows for quicker access to judicially approved wiretaps. It makes it compulsory for callers to disclose who they are, the purpose of the call and those on whose behalf they are calling. It makes it an offence to offer any prize for which the winner must pay cash up front.

The banks have also become involved in fraud awareness programs in Canada. They have mounted an educational program entitled *The ABC's of Fraud*, which has been given to many seniors groups across Canada (Henderson, 1997). Health Canada has also published a pamphlet on financial abuse of older adults that is widely distributed (Health Canada, 1999).

Many provincial governments and organizations have been active in educating consumers and seniors about consumer fraud. For instance, the Ministry of Consumer Affairs in Ontario in partnership with other government agencies and businesses has put out a Fraud Free calendar for five years (Ministry of Consumer & Business Services, 2002). It features important information every month about frequent scams and is targeted at seniors.

Many local police departments put on education sessions for seniors and those who serve vulnerable seniors such as Meals on Wheels or Homecare programs. The Better Business Bureau also helps arrange seminars to local seniors groups. In Toronto, Ontario, a strategic partnership has developed between the Toronto police, Ontario Provincial Police, provincial government, Competition bureau, United States Federal Trade Commission, and the United States Postal Service to combat fraudulent telemarketing (Cribb et al., 2002).

They have reportedly shut down 42 operators since February 2002 but there is still concern about sentencing of those prosecuted.

Recommendations have been made to Canadian physicians (see above) about the prevention of elder abuse in general (Canadian Task Force). Krueger et al. explored strategies that family physicians could employ in dealing with elder abuse in Canada. They asked the physicians in their study to rate eleven potential strategies. Those the physicians said they were fairly or very likely to use included: call an agency regarding the care (95%), consult a directory of services for seniors (90%) or list of resource people for advice on elder abuse (87%), elder abuse resource package or professional guidelines for detection and management of elder abuse (83%). The research group proposes to work to prepare algorithms to help physicians in the future when they suspect elder abuse. Cohen has recommended that physicians think about their patients who are older, female, socially isolated, and cognitively impaired as potential victims of consumer fraud (Cohen, 2002). Cohen recommends that physicians ask these patients about financial arrangements such as power of attorney and if possible notify their families about potential abuse. Physicians can also access important information about how to spot victims of telemarketing fraud on the PhoneBusters website (*www.phonebusters.com*).

CONCLUSIONS

Consumer fraud is an ongoing concern in Canada and seniors represent a disproportionate percentage of victims. Many organizations have responded to this challenge and Canada has seen the development of unique educational materials and diverse national, provincial and local strategies, particularly in the area of telemarketing fraud. Recent police initiatives and changes in the law will hopefully lead to stricter sentences for offenders and this may reduce the incentive for some types of crime. Much research remains to be done on the prevalence of consumer fraud, the consequences for the victims and the many types of fraud schemes that are being used. However, education of seniors, identification of those at risk of abuse and recognition of victims will continue to be important methods of preventing the devastating effects of these crimes in the future.

REFERENCES

Bailey, S. (1999, Jul. 12). Postal carrier suspended: She won't deliver 'scam' cards. *The Toronto Star*, p. A4.

Canadian Association of Retired Persons, (1999). CARP Bulletins: Getting tough on Fraud. *CARP News*, August 1999, p. 11.

Canadian Task Force on the Periodic Health Examination. Periodic health examination, 1994 update: 4 (1994). Secondary prevention of elder abuse and mistreatment. *CMAJ,* 151, 1413-1420.

Cohen, C.A. (2002). Consumer Fraud and the Vulnerable Older Adult. *Annals of the Royal College of Physicians and Surgeons of Canada,* 35(6), 354-356.

Cribb, R., & Cotroneo, C. (2002 Nov. 4). In telemarketing world, Canada is the Wild West. *The Toronto Star,* p. A8.

Health Canada, Government of Canada (1999). *Financial Abuse of Older Adults.* Cat. H72-22/8-1998E, ISBN 0-662-27401-6.

Henderson, H. (1997, Nov. 29) Troupe helps seniors recognize a fraud artist. *The Toronto Star,* p. M3.

Krueger, P., & Patterson, C. (1997). Detecting and managing elder abuse: Challenges in primary care. *Can Med Assoc Journal,* 157(8), 1095-1100.

MacAulay, J. (1998). If it's not someone you trust . . . Learn to say 'NO.' *CARP News,* August 1998, vol. 14 (4).

Mascoll, P. (1999, Apr. 24). Record sentence for telephone fraud. *The Toronto Star,* p. B4.

McDonald, P.L., Hornick, J.P., Robertson, G. B., & Wallace, J.E. (1991). *Elder Abuse and Neglect in Canada.* Butterworths, Toronto, 17.

Ministry of Consumer & Business Services, Government of Ontario (2002). Fraud Free Calendar 2002, www.cbs.gov.on.ca, 1-800-889-9768.

Muggeridge, P. (1999). CARP takes aim at con artists, *CARP News,* August 1999, vol. 15, p. 06.

National Advisory Council on Aging, Government of Canada (2001). Expression, Bulletin of the National Advisory Council on Aging, Spring 2001. ISSN 0922-8213, 14(2).

Otiniano, M.E., Lorimor, R., & MacDonald, E. (1998). Seniors targeted by fraud. *The Gerontologist Special Issue* (October) 38, 306.

PhoneBusters, *www.phonebusters.com,* 1-888-495-8501.

Podnieks, E. (1992). National survey on abuse of the elderly in Canada. *Journal of Elder Abuse & Neglect,* 4(5), 58.

Vida, S. (1994). An update on elder abuse and neglect. *Canadian Journal of Psychiatry,* 39 Supplement 1: S34-S40.

Psycho-Educational Support Groups for Older Women Victims of Family Mistreatment: A Pilot Study

Patricia Brownell, PhD
Deborah Heiser, PhD

SUMMARY. Few programs for domestic violence victims have been evaluated for effectiveness. This gap is even more pronounced for elder abuse service interventions. The study presented here is intended to address this gap by using an experimental research design to evaluate outcomes of an elder mistreatment psycho-social support group pilot for cognitively unimpaired older female victims of mistreatment by family members and significant others for whom they are providing care or support. The support group model used for the study adapts a model designed by NOVA House, an elder abuse shelter program in Manitoba, Canada. The study was funded by the Hartford Foundation Geriatric Social Work Faculty Scholars Program. While the significance of study findings is limited by the small number of pilot participants, the model intervention and evaluation instrument developed for the study may be utilized for study replication. *[Article copies available for a fee from The Haworth Document Delivery Service: 1-800-HAWORTH. E-mail address: <docdelivery@haworthpress. com> Website: <http://www.HaworthPress.com> © 2006 by The Haworth Press, Inc. All rights reserved.]*

[Haworth co-indexing entry note]: "Psycho-Educational Support Groups for Older Women Victims of Family Mistreatment: A Pilot Study." Brownell, Patricia, and Deborah Heiser. Co-published simultaneously in *Journal of Gerontological Social Work* (The Haworth Press, Inc.) Vol. 46, No. 3/4, 2006, pp. 145-160 ; and: *Elder Abuse and Mistreatment: Policy, Practice, and Research* (ed: M. Joanna Mellor, and Patricia Brownell) The Haworth Press, Inc., 2006, pp. 145-160. Single or multiple copies of this article are available for a fee from The Haworth Document Delivery Service [1-800-HAWORTH, 9:00 a.m. - 5:00 p.m. (EST). E-mail address: docdelivery@haworthpress.com].

KEYWORDS. Elder abuse, psycho-educational support group intervention, gerontology, older women, family mistreatment

PROBLEM STATEMENT

Elder mistreatment is a social problem that has received increasing recognition in recent years (Wolf, 2000). It is defined as physical, psychological, and financial abuse, and neglect of an older adult at least 60 years of age by a family member, friend, or acquaintance (Wolf & Pillemer, 1984). Estimates of prevalence rates range from 4-10 percent (Pillemer & Finkelhor, 1988; U. S. House of Representatives, 1990). The 1998 National Incidence Report estimated incidence of elder abuse as 1.9 percent (NCEA, 1998), which is considered low by some experts in the field.

The current demographics of population aging in the United States suggest that the adult population aged 60 years and older will continue to increase as the baby boomers (those born between 1946 and 1964) reach old age (Federal Interagency Forum on Aging-Related Statistics, 2000). If the percentage of older people who are abused by family members remains stable, the numbers of elder abuse victims can be expected to increase as well.

Women are especially challenged in the process of successful aging because of a number of factors, including inequities in financial resources, the assumption of family caregiving responsibilities, and societal ageism that celebrates youth over maturity (Garner, 1999). In addition, the widespread abuse of women of all ages has been well-documented (Vinton, 1999). This includes older women, who have been reported as vulnerable to abuse by adult children (Brownell, 1998), as well as partners and spouses.

Early studies of elder mistreatment suggested that care dependent older adults were most likely to be abused by overwhelmed caregivers (Steinmetz, 1988). Other studies, notably a large scale prevalence study conducted in Boston, challenged the findings of these early studies (Pillemer & Finkelhor, 1988), suggesting instead that caregiving older adults were most at risk of abuse by those impaired family members for whom they were providing care.

According to Bergeron (2001), theories that practitioners hold about the etiology of social problems of clients they serve shape their practice in the field. Those practitioners who believe that elder abuse is associated with caregiver stress may support interventions that provide relief to caregivers of care dependent older adults. Respite services, caregiver support groups, and use of formal services to supplement informal family care are examples of service interventions that evolve from this theoretical orientation. Elder abuse victims who do not match this profile of frail and care dependent older adults may be overlooked by these practitioners.

Proponents of abuser impairment or deviance as associated with elder abuse may advocate for interventions that draw on the legal and criminal justice system. Practitioners who work with older abused women may be unsure as to whether to engage domestic violence or aging service networks as part of their interventions (Vinton, 1999). In addition, practitioners have noted that older victims of family abuse often resist interventions that they believe may harm their abuser, and often deny the seriousness of the abuse.

This response pattern is well-known in the field of domestic violence, where victims may resist or deny abuse by spouses or partners. While remedies exist in the criminal justice system, domestic violence victims may choose not to utilize them. Reasons include concern for the well-being of the abuser, fear of the abuser, lack of understanding about the dynamics of domestic violence, sense of social isolation, and lack of knowledge about the range of remedies and coping strategies that may be available.

For elder abuse victims, or victims of family mistreatment, barriers to obtaining services may include physical and cognitive frailty, and dependence on the abuser. However, victims may also serve in a caregiving or support capacity to their dependent, abusive family members, creating different but nonetheless challenging barriers to the victims' acceptance of needed services for themselves (Brownell, Berman, & Salamone, 1999). Remedies such as legal guardianships and other protective services intended for the mentally and physically impaired adults (Quinn & Tomita, 1997) are not appropriate or available for cognitively unimpaired elder abuse victims. Crisis or empowerment oriented services may not be available to unimpaired older women who are victims of family mistreatment.

The dynamics of domestic violence or family mistreatment can continue into old age as a pattern of coercive control that one family member exercises over another through physical violence, threats, emotional insults, and economic deprivation (Schechter, 1982). However, the issues that must be confronted by older women who are abused or mistreated are complicated by the dynamics of families in later life and the normal tasks of aging (Vinton, 1999).

In the domestic violence field, the psycho-educational support group has been used as an intervention for women who are domestic violence victims (Podnieks, 1999). However, this model is not commonly available to older women who may be abused by impaired family members for whom they are providing care or support, and may require adaptation to the special needs of older women who are victims of family mistreatment.

Few programs for domestic violence victims have been evaluated for effectiveness using sound research methods (Chalk & King, 1998). This gap is even more pronounced for elder abuse service interventions. A study by the National Research Institute found that only two evaluations of elder abuse programs met the standard for sound evaluative research as defined by the Committee on the Assessment of Family Violence Intervention, convened in 1994 to assess the gap between research resources and policy needs related to addressing the problem of domestic violence, including elder abuse (Chalk & King, 1998). In addition, no evaluations to date have been undertaken for elder mistreatment psycho-educational support group models as an intervention strategy.

The study presented here is intended to address the gap between research resources and policy needs by evaluating the outcome of an elder mistreatment psycho-social support group model for cognitively unimpaired older female victims of mistreatment by family members and significant others for whom they are providing care or support. External outcome objectives for support group participants were: Increase in social network and increase in locus of control (efficacy). Internal outcome objectives for support group participants were: Increase in self-esteem, decrease in depression, decrease in anxiety and somatization, and decrease in guilt. The support group model used for the study replicates a model designed by NOVA House, an elder abuse shelter program in Manitoba, Canada (Schmuland, 1995). The study was funded by the Hartford Foundation Geriatric Social Work Faculty Scholars Program.

RESEARCH QUESTIONS

1. Does a psycho-educational support group make a difference for older women (age 60 years and older) who are victims of family mistreatment?
2. As compared with a control group, do older women who participate in an 8-week, 2 hour session per week, elder mistreatment psycho-educational support group demonstrate the following:

- Increased sense of control (measured by Health Locus of Control Scale)?
- Increased sense of social support (measured by Medical Outcomes Study Social Support Survey)?
- Decreased depression (measured by CES-D 10)?
- Decreased anxiety and somatization (measured by BSI-18)?
- Increased self-esteem (measured by Rosenberg Self-Esteem Scale)?
- Decreased guilt (measured by Guilt subscale in Multi-Problem Screening Inventory)?

The study was also intended to develop a socio-demographic profile of victims of elder mistreatment who are candidates for participation in support group interventions. This included race/ethnicity; age; income; educational level; marital status; living situation; work history and status; religious affiliation; relationship with abuser; history of abuse with identified abuser; physical and emotional functioning (measured by SF-36 Physical Functioning (PF) Scale and Rand-36 Role Physical (RP) Scale; SF-36 Role-Emotional (RE) Scale; SF-36 Social Functioning (SF) Scale; SF-36 General Health (GH) Scale); religiosity (as measured by Duke University Religion Scale); substance use (measured by SMAST-G; Drug Use sub-scale: Multi-Problem Screening Inventory); type and intensity of abuse experienced (measured by abuse sub-scales: Multi-Problem Screening Inventory); attendance at elder mistreatment psycho-educational support group sessions (measured by attendance log for those study participants randomly assigned to the intervention); and suicidality (measured by Suicidality Sub-Scale: Multi-Problem Screening Inventory).

SIGNIFICANCE OF STUDY

Elder abuse support groups are recommended as effective interventions for older victims of family mistreatment (Podnieks, 1999; Seaver, 1996). In one study, older victims of family mistreatment identified support groups as one of a few services they would accept if offered (Brownell, Berman, & Salamone, 1999). However, little is known about the effectiveness of this treatment modality (Wolf, 1998; Chalk & King, 1998).

To date, the most comprehensive study of elder abuse support groups was undertaken by the late Rosalie Wolf, who completed a descriptive study of elder abuse support groups in the United States in 1998. Dr. Wolf identified two types of support group providers: domestic violence and aging. Podnieks (2002), in a discussion of elder abuse focus and support groups from an international perspective, identified elder abuse support groups as having a number of psychosocial benefits. These include: developing mutual support relationship with peers that supplement depleted natural networks; moving beyond guilt; enhancing self-esteem; and learning problem-solving and coping strategies.

Dr. Podnieks acknowledges that these benefits are identified based on anecdotal evidence, and small provider and client satisfaction surveys. More information is needed on how support groups benefit elder abuse victims, and who benefits more than others. This is timely as there is increasing interest in elder abuse as a public health, criminal justice, and aging issue. The World

Health Organization (WHO) has funded a multi-national study on elder abuse in developing and developed countries (Dr. Gerry Bennett, Personal Communication, October 10, 2002).

The Elder Justice Bill (Breaux-Hatch, 2004) proposed funding for elder abuse services and research. The Violence Against Women's Act (VAWA) 2000 has a section on enhancing protections for older women from domestic violence and sexual assault. On the local level in New York City, the New York City Department for the Aging (DFTA) has contracted with selected community partners to provide services, including support groups, to elder abuse victims in the community (Aurora Salamone, Director, Elderly Crime Victims Resource Unit, New York City Department for the Aging, Personal Communication, December 1, 2004).

The findings of the pilot study can provide valuable information on model building and testing one approach to serving elder abuse victims through a psycho-educational support group intervention. In the planning of this pilot study, the Principal Investigator (P.I.) worked closely with DFTA's Research and Elderly Crime Victims Resource units, as well as aging service providers in New York City who have received or are interested in applying for funds from DFTA to implement service programs, including support groups, for elder abuse victims in their communities. Study findings can also inform the international community through dissemination of information at conferences, and in journals and newsletters.

METHODOLOGY

The support group sessions were held at the Fordham University Graduate School of Social Service. Pre and post study interviews were conducted for both control and intervention group participants at the agencies of community partners, and Fordham University.

The sample included sixteen (16) women age 69 to 83 identified by participating community partners as meeting the criteria for the study and agreed to participate. Nine were randomly assigned to the intervention group and 6 were randomly assigned to the control group. Eligibility criteria for study participation included: Self-identified to an aging service provider as having family problems that include family member behaviors associated with physical, psychological, and/or financial abuse; no significant cognitive impairment, based on assessments of professional social workers serving as aging provider referral sources; able to communicate in English; connected to an aging service provider with the capability to provide crisis intervention and additional needed services; and able and willing to attend a weekly support group meeting, 2 hours in length, for 8 consecutive weeks.

The support group curriculum included content on domestic violence and older women (session one); abuse and neglect of older women (session two); the legacies of troubled families (session three); assessing family histories (session four); enhancing self-esteem (session five); dealing with depression, anxiety and stress, substance abuse, and gambling (session six); coping with loss and change in relationships with loved ones and strategies for change (session seven); and service resources and closure (session eight). Refer to Table 1 for Support Group Curriculum.

Intervention: The intervention was *a 2-hour psycho-educational support group, held weekly for 8 consecutive weeks.* A retired professional social worker and a graduate social work student facilitated the group sessions.

OUTREACH

Outreach was initiated to professional social work aging service providers who may have contact with older women at least 60 years of age who are victims of elder mistreatment as a form of domestic violence was conducted in partnership with the New York City Department for the Aging (DFTA). Service providers who agreed to participate in the study screening and referral process included the DFTA Elderly Crime Victims Resource Center, the DFTA Grandparents Resource Center, senior centers, elderly crime victims programs, the NYC Human Resources Administration (HRA) Domestic Violence Program, and the HRA Adult Protective Services Program.

DATA COLLECTION

Data for the study were collected in two ways. As part of the evaluation, in-person, pre- and post-intervention interviews were conducted two months before and after the intervention period with each study participant, including both intervention and control group participants. Each interview lasted approximately one hour, and included socio-demographics as well as measures for social network support, locus of control, depression, anxiety and somatization, guilt, substance use, religiosity, and type and intensity of abuse. While data were also collected through audiotapes of each support group session, to identify themes, and relationship between support group content and group

TABLE 1. Curriculum for Support Group

Session 1 Domestic Violence and Older Women	Session 2 Abuse and Neglect of Older Women	Session 3 The Legacies of Troubled Families	Session 4 The Silver Cord: Family History	Session 5 Enhancing Self-Esteem	Session 6 Depression, Anxiety and Stress: Feeling Bad About Ourselves; Drug, Alcohol, and Gambling Addictions	Session 7 Coping with Loss and Changes in Relationships with Loved Ones and Strategies for Change	Session 8 Closing Session
45 min.– Introduce session	15 min.– Introduce session	30 min. – Introduce session	30 min.– Introduce session	30 min.– 3 Tasks	10 min.– Present depression handouts	20 min.– Present handouts and complete activity 1	
30 min.– video: "Elder Abuse: 5 case studies"	35 min. – video: "A House Divided: Caregiver Stress and Elder Abuse"	45 min.– 3 group activities with group exercises	30 min.– 3 group activities	25 min.– synopsis of video activity 1	10 min.– discuss issues raised	10 min.– video synopsis	
20 min.– discuss video	10 min.– discuss video	23 min.– video and synopsis: "Adult Children of Alcoholics"	10 min.– video and synopsis: "Just to Have a Peaceful Life"	10 min.– discuss video	10 min.– closing round	10 min.– present and complete activity	
10 min.– closing round	45 min.– overview of Valued Traits and Vulnerabilities	15 min.– discuss video	30 min.– discuss video	20 min.– complete activity 2 with group	20 min.– present materials and complete activity 1	20 min.– overview of services and interventions	
	10 min.– summary	5 min.– closing round	25 min.– closing round	5 min.– closing round	10 min.– discuss issues	20 min.– role play	
	5 min.– closing round			20 min.– Present material	30 min.– Present drinking, drugs, and gampling handouts	10 min.– reflect on lessons learned	
				15 min.– synopsis of video	10 min.– discuss issues raised		
				10 min.– discuss video	5 min.– closing round		
				5 min.– closing round			

member responses, this article will report on selected evaluation data collected in the pre and post interviews with study subjects.

Data were collected using an evaluation instrument developed for the study. In addition to factual questions regarding information categories listed above, it also included scales to evaluate intervention outcomes. Scales imbedded in the instrument included the CES-D Depression Scale, the Rosenberg Self-Esteem Scale, the Duke Religiosity Scale, the Hudson Substance Use Scale, the BSI, Hudson Multi-problem Symptom Inventory (MPSI), the Social Support Scale, and the Locus of Control Scale. Some of these measures, such as the Rosenberg Self-Esteem Scale, the Social Support Scale, and the CES-D Depression Scale, have been used in evaluations of other domestic violence and elder abuse programs (Chalk & King, 1998).

DATA ANALYSIS

Interview measures were compared within and between groups to determine whether changes occurred and could be identified by comparing before and after scores for the intervention group, and between intervention and control groups, using non-parametric statistical analysis. While the small sample size precludes the possibility of obtaining statistically significant findings, it is anticipated that the findings of the pilot study will contribute to the development of a model for ongoing evaluation of elder mistreatment support groups, and some suggestion of a direction as to the effectiveness of the support group model being evaluated.

FINDINGS

Description of Sample

There was no statistical difference between the control and intervention group participants, examining socio-demographic characteristics of group participants.

Age: The average age of the 16 participants was 75-years-old: the youngest was 68 and the oldest was 83.

Race/Ethnicity: Both groups included 50% White, 44% Black, and 6% Asian/ Pacific Islander (control group) or Hispanic (intervention group). The majority of study participants were born in the United States (69%), with 12.5% in Central/South America, 12.5% in Europe, and 6% in Asia.

Marital Status/Living Arrangements: Collectively, 12.5% were married, 12.5% were living together, 25% were separated, 25% were divorced, and 25% were widowed. The average length of time in the current marital status was 22 years. The majority of participants (56%) had two people living in the home, while 25% had one, 12.5% had three, and 6% had four. Nearly 90% of the participants lived in their own home/apartment, while approximately 12% lived with relatives or boarded with nonrelatives/nonfriends. The average length of stay in their current residence was 17 years, and ranged from less than one month to 46 years.

Insurance: The vast majority received Medicare and Medicaid, 94% and 81% respectively, and 81% had another kind of health insurance that paid bills in addition to Medicare/Medicaid. More than 80% of the participants reported they never lacked the kind of medical care they should have, while 19% reported they lacked needed medical care once in awhile.

Education: The average level of education completed was 13 years with the lowest level being 7 years and the highest 19 years.

Finances: The majority (72%) had a total household income less than $20,000 while for 19%, income ranged between $35,000 and $50,000. For 6% income was more than $50,000. Nearly 40% of the participants felt they did not have enough money to make ends meet at the end of the month, while 30% felt they had just enough and 30% had some money left over.

Religion: Participants were mostly Catholic (38%), while 31% were Protestant, 25% were Jewish, and 6% (one) reported no religious affiliation.

Work Status: The vast majority (81%) were not working at a paying job. Of the 19% who worked, 13% worked part-time and 6% worked 35 hours per week. Most (88%) were retired and had been for an average of 26 years. The majority (81%) did not volunteer at non-paying jobs.

Relationship with Family Abuser: The majority of participants (62.5%) identified an adult son as their abuser, 25% identified a spouse, and 6% identified a daughter and a nephew, respectively.

BEHAVIORAL TRAITS

Behavioral traits measured in the study included alcohol use, drug (including prescription drug) use, perceptions of family relations problems, relationships between victims and abusers, and type of abuse experienced. There were no statistically significant differences within or between the two groups of study participants (control and intervention) on these measures.

Alcohol Abuse: Based on the Short Michigan Alcoholism Screening Test (SMAST-G), 31% of controls and 6% of intervention participants suffered from an alcohol problem.

Drug Use: The majority (100% of controls and 89% of intervention participants) did not have a problem with drug abuse. One intervention participant was identified as having a potential problem with prescription drug use, based on the scale used in the study.

Family Relations: The majority (60% of controls and 78% of intervention participants) had family relationship problems, based on the Hartford Family Relationship Problems Subscale.

Types of Abuse Experienced: The majority, 83% of controls and 100% of intervention subjects, reported non-physical abuse, based on the Hartford Study Non-physical Abuse Subscale. Based on the Hartford Study Physical Abuse Subscale, 43% of controls and 22% of intervention participants reported physical abuse.

Suicide: None of the participants were suicidal according to the Hartford Suicide Subscale.

OUTCOME MEASURES

Participants did not differ within or between groups on the identified outcome measures utilized in the study. These included: depression, guilt, and self-esteem. There were no significant changes in these measures for either control or intervention group participants after the intervention ended.

Depression: Based on the CESB-D 10, 14% of controls and 56% of intervention participants suffered from depression.

Guilt: According to the Hartford Study Guilt Subscale, 28% of the control participants scored above threshold and 33% of the intervention participants scored above threshold.

Self-Esteem: Results from the Rosenberg Self-Esteem Scale (range is 10 to 40) indicated that participants scored an average of 32, which is above the midpoint (see Table 2).

DISCUSSION

As may be expected, the socio-demographic profile of study participants reflects a relatively unimpaired and high functioning cohort of elder mistreatment victims. This is because of the eligibility criteria for an elder mistreatment psycho-educational support group for community-dwelling victims.

TABLE 2. Outcome Measures Pre and Post Intervention

	Alcohol Abuse	Depression	Drug Use	Family Relations Problems	Guilt	Suicide	Non-phys. Abuse	Phys. Abuse
Control Pre-test	31%	14%	0	60%	28%	0	83%	43%
Intervention Pre-test	6%	56%	11%	78%	33%	0	100%	22%
Control Pre-test and Intervention Pre-test	$p = .90$	$p = .37$	$p = .37$	$p = .52$	$p = .76$	n/a	$p = .67$	$p = .33$
Control Post-test	23%	33%	0	100%	14%	0	75%	0
Intervention Post-test	6%	56%	0	86%	22%	0	83%	13%
Control Post-test and Intervention Post-test	$p = .66$	$p = .49$	$p = .37$	$p = .22$	$p = .72$	n/a	$p = .75$	$p = .41$
Control Pre-test and Control Post-test	$p = 1.0$	$p = 1.0$	$p = .37$	$p = .32$	$p = .95$	n/a	$p = .59$	$p = .09$
Intervention Pre-test and Intervention Post-test	$p = .78$	$p = .91$	$p = .34$	$p = .88$	$p = .5$	n/a	$p = .48$	$p = .58$

Criteria necessarily will screen out prospective participants who are assessed as having a high degree of cognitive or psychiatric impairment, due to the demands of this treatment model for participant capacity for group interaction, and information retention and processing.

However, the profile also challenges a perception of elder mistreatment victims that suggests they experience low self-esteem, lack of a social network support, fragile mental status, and dependency on family members for basic necessities like food, medical care, and housing. This cohort of sixteen (16) victims had relatively high self-esteem, sometimes extensive social network supports, exhibited some depression and anxiety but no suicidality, and relatively little drug and alcohol abuse, and had access to medical care through Medicare or Medicaid. Most lived in their own homes or apartments, and few identified problems obtaining sufficient food to eat. They identified themselves overall as a moderately religious group, and while most had relatively low incomes, all had some income through pensions, social security, employment, and in one case Supplemental Security Income (SSI). All were identified as having problem families, which is not surprising since experience of family abuse was one criterion for participation in the study.

Comparing their scores with *Key Indicators of Well-Being*, a national study on health (Federal Interagency Forum on Aging Related Statistics, 2000), and *Alcoholism: Getting the Facts* (National Institute on Alcohol Abuse and Alcoholism, 2004), participants presented as more depressed, more likely to use alcohol and slightly less likely to experience illnesses associated with age but slightly more likely to identify themselves as experiencing poorer health than others their age. However, overall they appeared not to differ significantly on socio-demographic measures from others in their age cohort.

Control and intervention group members did not differ significantly on socio-demographic or behavioral measures like substance abuse, suicidality, religiosity, family problems, depression and anxiety, and family problems and abuse. Thus, any change on outcome measures of interest in the study (depression, anxiety and somatization, locus of control, perception of social network support, guilt, and self-esteem) could be attributed to the effects of the group as opposed to differences between the control and intervention group member characteristics.

Analysis of outcomes associated with the group intervention revealed no change for either control or intervention groups. In other words, there was no significant difference between control and intervention groups before and after the elder mistreatment psycho-educational support group intervention on any of the outcome measures hypothesized to be influenced by the support group experience, based on the measures used in the study. This is in spite of the self-reports of the intervention group members. All but one of the group members identified the group as helpful in increasing their self-esteem and feelings of well-being. The dissenting group member believed that the group content should be more focused on concrete problem-solving and positive visions for the future.

IMPLICATIONS FOR FURTHER RESEARCH

The study did not find any change in the hypothesized outcome measures for study participants, calling into question the effectiveness of the psycho-educational support group model for increasing the well-being of elder abuse victim participants. However, there may be alternative explanations for these findings. First, the sample size was very small (a total of 16 participants). Larger numbers of participants and groups would need to be studied to come to a conclusion about the effectiveness of this intervention model. Second, the measures used for the study may not be appropriate or sensitive enough to evaluate outcomes (either beneficial or not). Third, some of the assumptions in the literature on which the study was based may be inaccurate. Fourth, participants may benefit from longer group sessions (i.e., 12 weeks or more). Finally, participants were receiving social service support prior to the start of the study, which may have had an impact on the study: (1) those who were already receiving support may have higher self-esteem and differ in their socio-demographic profile compared with the population; and (2) they may be qualitatively different from those who did not seek/accept the support.

The socio-demographic and behavioral profile of women who participated in the group does not reflect that of the commonly accepted profile of elder abuse victims in the literature, even in the literature on support groups. This group of 16 women had high self-esteem, relatively low depression, relatively strong social network supports, and a relatively high degree of self-sufficiency before the intervention began.

Since the support group intervention was assumed to make a difference in these measures, based on assumptions about the target population that was not found to be accurate, perhaps different measures should be used to assess effectiveness in the future. Also, it suggests that either this was an atypical group of subjects, or that more information is needed about the psycho-social status of this cohort of older woman abuse victims before more effective interventions can be designed and tested.

Institutional Review Board issues: University-based research on elder abuse faces a number of ethical and methodological challenges (Dresser, 2003). Concerns on the part of University institutional review boards (IRBs) charged with the responsibility for ensuring the protection of human research subjects, particularly those identified as vulnerable, places limitations on the level of research inquiry into the social problem of elder abuse. In the study described here, the Fordham University IRB felt strongly that to ensure adequate protection for participating elder abuse victims, safeguards needed to be in place to ensure that their safety and well-being was maximized. As a result, one requirement for the study was that each study participant be served by a social worker in an agency setting during the course of the study.

A second requirement was that all subjects continue to receive social services through their identified social work and social service agency, so the intervention studied was an additional service. The levels of service subjects received in addition to the psycho-educational support group intervention was a variable for which that the researcher could not control. Because agency records are confidential, and a waiver of confidentiality was not sought in this research project, the concurrent services any given subject might have been receiving were not included in the study design.

Serious ethical concerns would likely arise for any research project on psycho-educational support groups conducted in the community that attempted to prevent subjects from obtaining additional services available to them. However, by including a measure of these concurrent services, subsequent outcome studies could help to identify an interactional effect, if any, among the intervention of interest and other interventions, if any, that subjects received concurrently.

CONCLUSION

The pilot study presented here was among the first to examine the effectiveness of an elder mistreatment psycho-educational support group model under experimental conditions, using subjects randomly assigned to control and intervention groups, and outcomes measured through pre and post tests. The study found no change in hypothesized outcomes between the control and intervention groups. Because of the small sample size of the study (a total of sixteen participants), findings are not conclusive and further research is needed.

Of interest is the information on the profile of the study subjects that challenges assumptions about the cohort of elder mistreatment victims that could benefit from a psycho-educational support group intervention. The subjects that volunteered to participate in the study had high self-esteem, as a group had relatively well-developed social networks, were in relatively good health for their age cohort, and were relatively self-sufficient. The socio-demographic and other measures used in the study did not differentiate these elder abuse victims from other older women in their age cohort. This in turn suggests that risk factors for elder abuse victimization are not intrinsic to the victim herself.

More research is needed on profiles of victimization as well as effectiveness of intervention strategies for different sub-populations of elder abuse victims.

REFERENCES

Bergeron, L. R. (2001). An elder abuse case study: Caregiver stress or domestic violence? You decide. *Journal of Gerontological Social Work,* 34, *4,* 47-63.

Brownell, P. (1998). *Family crimes against the elderly: Elder abuse and the criminal justice system.* New York: Garland Publishing Company.

Brownell, P., Berman, J., and Salamone, A. (1999). Mental health and criminal justice issues among perpetrators of elder abuse. *Journal of Elder Abuse & Neglect,* 11, *4,* 81-94.

Chalk, R., and King, P.A. (1998). *Violence in families: Assessing prevention and treatment programs.* Washington, DC: National Research Council and Institute of Medicine.

Dresser, R. (2003). *Ethical and policy issue in research in elder abuse and neglect.* In National Research Council, *Elder Mistreatment: Abuse, Neglect, and Exploitation in an Aging America.* Washington, DC: The National Academies Press.

Federal Interagency Forum on Aging-Related Statistics (2000). *Key indicators of well-being.* Washington: DC.

Garner, D. (1999). Feminism and feminist gerontology. In Garner, D. (Ed.), *Fundamentals of Feminist Gerontology.* Binghamton, NY: The Haworth Press, Inc., 3-12.

National Center on Elder Abuse (1998). *The national elder abuse incidence study*. Washington, DC: United States Department of Health and Human Services/Administration/Administration on Aging.

National Institute on Alcohol Abuse and Alcoholism (NIAAA). *Alcoholism: Getting the facts*. Retrieved from the World Wide Web on September 14, 2004 *http://www.niaaa.nih.gov/publications/booklet.htm*

Pillemer, K., and Finkelhor, D. (1988). The prevalence of elder abuse: A random sample survey. *The Gerontologist*, 28, *1*, 51-57.

Podnieks, E. (2002). *Focus groups in the abuse and neglect of older adults*. Unpublished manuscript.

Podnieks, E. (1999). Support groups: A chance at human connections for abused older adults. In Prichard, J. (Ed.), *Elder Abuse Work: Best Practice in Britain and Canada*. London: Jessica Kingsley Publishers, 457-483.

Quinn, M. J., and Tomita, S. (1997). *Elder abuse and neglect: Causes, diagnosis, and intervention strategies*, 2nd Edition. New York: Springer Publishing Company.

Schechter, S. (1982). *Women and male violence: The visions and struggles of the battered women's movement*. Boston, MA: South End Press.

Schmuland, F. (1995). *Shelter support groups for abused older women: A facilitator's manual*. Selkirk, Manitoba: Nova House Women's Shelter.

Seaver, C. (1996). Muted lives: Older battered women. *Journal of Elder Abuse & Neglect*, 8, *2*, 3-21.

Steinmetz, S. (1980). *Duty bound*. Newbury Park, CA: Sage Publishing Company.

U.S. House of Representatives (1990). *Elder abuse: Decade of shame and inaction*. Washington, DC: United States Government Printing Office.

Vinton, L. (1999). Working with abused older women from a feminist perspective. In Garner, D. (Ed.), *Fundamentals of Feminist Gerontology*. Binghamton, NY: The Haworth Press, Inc.

Wolf, R. S. (1998). *Support groups for older victims of domestic violence: Sponsors and programs*. Washington, DC: National Committee for the Prevention of Elder Abuse, Grant Number 90-AM-0660.

Wolf, R. S., and Pillemer, K. (1984). *Definitions of elder abuse and neglect*. New York: New York City Elder Abuse Coalition.

RESEARCH

Ethical and Psychosocial Issues Raised by the Practice in Cases of Mistreatment of Older Adults

Marie Beaulieu, PhD
Nancy Leclerc, Social Worker, MA

SUMMARY. Intervention regarding older adult mistreatment raises many questions for practitioners. They have to interact with the victim, the abuser, and, in many cases, with both of them at the same time. In such cases, five themes emerge from the literature review on psycho-social and ethical issues in practice: practitioners' pre-construction and axiological frameworks, victims' capacity, confidentiality versus collaboration between practitioners or between agencies, social and family responsibilities and the balance between competing values in practice. Practitioners are well placed to offer a critical reflection on their practice and on ways of improving it. The goal of our qualitative study is to iden-

[Haworth co-indexing entry note]: "Ethical and Psychosocial Issues Raised by the Practice in Cases of Mistreatment of Older Adults." Beaulieu, Marie, and Nancy Leclerc. Co-published simultaneously in *Journal of Gerontological Social Work* (The Haworth Press, Inc.) Vol. 46, No. 3/4, 2006, pp. 161-186 ; and: *Elder Abuse and Mistreatment: Policy, Practice, and Research* (ed: M. Joanna Mellor, and Patricia Brownell) The Haworth Press, Inc., 2006, pp. 161-186. Single or multiple copies of this article are available for a fee from The Haworth Document Delivery Service [1-800-HAWORTH, 9:00 a.m. - 5:00 p.m. (EST). E-mail address: docdelivery@haworthpress.com].

tify issues and ethical dilemmas in elderly mistreatment situations as represented in the discourses of practitioners in reference to interventions in their psychosocial practice. Sixteen practitioners from the public and community (non-profit organization) sectors were interviewed using a practice history approach. This paper presents the main ethical and psychosocial issues raised by practitioners and some ideas to improve the practice. It is motivated by the crucial question haunting the practitioners' minds: "How far should we go?" *[Article copies available for a fee from The Haworth Document Delivery Service: 1-800-HAWORTH. E-mail address: <docdelivery@haworthpress.com> Website: <http://www.HaworthPress. com> © 2006 by The Haworth Press, Inc. All rights reserved.]*

KEYWORDS. Mistreatment of older adults, intervention, ethical issues, psychosocial issues, values, practice improvement

INTRODUCTION

The nations of the world must create an environment in which ageing is accepted as a natural part of the life cycle, where anti-ageing attitudes are discouraged, where older people are given the right to live in dignity–free of abuse and exploitation–and are given opportunities to participate fully in educational, cultural, spiritual, and economic activities. (Randal & German, 1999, p. 143)

Research on mistreatment of older adults began in the 1970s. It has been decelerated by definitional, methodological, and theoretical problems. In fact, much research on the topic has been produced, yet it appears to be very difficult to obtain probing data on this issue; mistreatment tends to be kept more or less hidden. In the United States of America, programs administered by the Federal government on elder abuse are non-existent (Fulmer, 1991), and each state has its own protection laws (Bergeron, 2001). In Canada, legislation and practice vary according to provinces and territories (Beaulieu, Gordon, & Spencer, 2003). In Québec, where this study was conducted, protection laws for mistreated older adults do not exist, aside from a disposition on exploitation in the Provincial Charter of Rights.[1] It was only in the early 1980s that abuse and neglect began to be considered as a social problem (Beaulieu, 1992) or as a social dilemma (Spencer, 1998).

The seriousness and widespread problem of elder abuse affects approximately 700,000 to 1.2 million older adults on an annual basis in the United States of America. Reported figures are similar for Great Britain and Canada via sample surveys (Fulmer, 1998). In fact, two Canadian population studies have estimated that 4 to 7% of older adults living in the community are abused by persons they trust (Podnieks & Pillemer, 1990; Pottie Bunge, 2000). According to these statistics, material and financial exploitation is the most frequent form of abuse. Researchers agree that these statistics represent an underestimation of the magnitude of the problem.[2] Many cases of elder abuse are not reported (nine out of ten) and there is considerable underreporting by clinical professionals possibly due to inappropriate screening instruments (Fulmer, 2002).

Clinical practitioners (psychosocial and medical) are at the forefront for detecting elder abuse. Yet, they are often lacking the appropriate tools for the identification of abuse (accepted definition of elder abuse, nature and parameters of the problem) and intervention in such cases (limited knowledge base on elder abuse, lack of community support). They struggle with their own values, beliefs, and biases with regards to violence and the ageing family (Bookin & Dunkle, 1985). Individuals may be influenced by societal values conveyed around them, such as ageism or other beliefs on violence, family relationships, and so-on, whether they are practitioners or a member of an abuser-abused dyad.

Efficient action concerning mistreatment rests on the collaboration between professionals and services (Wolf & Pillemer, 1988; Spencer, 1998; Bergeron, 2001). This sense of renewal leads to a personal ethical self-reflection. Ethical positions may vary in accordance with professions and services. Not only is knowledge about violence and neglect important, but also experience and the willingness to consider each case as a unique intervention.

The purpose of this paper is to present the viewpoints of psychosocial practitioners on issues raised in their practice when working with cases of older adult mistreatment. They have plenty to share regarding values and actions, as well as psychosocial and ethical issues related to the practice. Based on their experience and on account of their focal position, they are well situated to recommend elements to enhance the guidelines and improve the practice. This article is divided as follows: review of the literature with regards to ethical and psychosocial issues raised by intervention in cases of older adult mistreatment, methodology, results and discussion, and conclusion. Our text is punctuated with quotes that illustrate the profundity of practitioners' concerns.

LITERATURE REVIEW

It is important that we continue to listen, learn, and be diligent in our efforts to tackle new challenges in ethical conduct. (Villani, 1994, p. 1)

Our literature review focuses on ethical and psychosocial issues related to practice with mistreated older adults. Therefore, it does not cover areas that are well documented such as victim characteristics, abuser characteristics, dynamics of abuse, legislation issues, impacts of abuse, social costs of abuse, different explanation theories, etc. One of the main issues when working in the field of older adult mistreatment is finding a common definition that everyone can agree upon. Many researchers and practitioners have proposed various definitions. At last, in 2002, The World Health Organization defined elder abuse by encompassing concerns of policy makers, practitioners and, more importantly, older adults themselves: *"Elder abuse is a single or repeated act, or lack of appropriate action, occurring within a relationship where there is an expectation of trust, which causes harm or distress to an older person. It can be of various forms: physical, psychological/emotional, sexual, financial, or simply reflect intentional or unintentional neglect"* (World Health Organization, 2002).

Our literature review has brought us to understand that even if many authors talk about psychosocial and ethical issues raised by the practice in cases of older adult mistreatment, very few are proposing results stemming from empirical research on ethical concerns. It appears that ethics is frequently treated as a reflexive account rather than as a subject-matter worthy of "serious" research.

Five themes emerge from the literature review. It is presented by an arrangement of ideas in a crescendo fashion. The first element, which is the reflection of one's own knowledge and one's own representations, is usually accessible to each and everyone. However, the last element, which involves an in-depth personal reflection on a person's way of doing and seeing things, is not within everyone's reach. The themes are (1) pre-construction and axiological framework, (2) victim's capacity, (3) confidentiality versus collaboration between professionals and services, (4) social or family responsibility, and (5) balance between competing values: autonomy, beneficence, non-malfeasance, and justice.

(1) Pre-Construction and Axiological Framework

In view of the fact that intervening in cases of older adult mistreatment raises confronting questions for practitioners on ageing, violence, personal relationships, and values, it is important for them to take the time to clarify their own position prior to being in contact with the victim or the abuser. Practitioners should perform an ethical self-reflection and question the values that they are putting forth when they intervene. Each older adult has his or her own values to be taken into consideration. Practitioners should not only be aware of them but should also honour them given that they are the most salient guidelines in the intervention process. This perspective may be idealistic, nevertheless, all practitioners should at least acknowledge and act in accordance with the values of older adults (Asch, 1993; Browdie, 1993; Dresser, 1993).

The representation practitioners have of the dynamics of mistreatment concerning older adults, along with their expertise in the field, determine their practice as well as their perception of the effectiveness of the interventions. A lack of knowledge or experience can lead to inactivity or a sense of pity for the elderly person (Saveman et al., 1997). In some cases, practitioners adopt a more neutral position, waiting for the situation to evolve instead of being proactive. In such cases, practitioners' inaction may generate emotions of distress within them. The complexity of the mistreatment situation creates feelings of failure, guilt or ineffectiveness (Saveman, 1992). The latter can provoke counter-transference; for instance, the practitioner will not agree to intervene as a result of the client's refusal, when in fact it is the practitioner's attitude during the intervention that brings the client to retreat (Bergeron, 1999).

(2) The Victims' Capacity

One of the first elements a practitioner ought to evaluate is the capacity for abused older adults to make their own decisions regarding their situation. In other words, mistreatment of older adults raises the question of autonomy. Practitioners must keep in mind that simply questioning the cognitive autonomy of the older adult or his/her capability is already an intrusion in one's lives. Ideally, they should avoid thinking that since they are intervening with an older person, he/she may be incapable. Should we not adopt a presumption of aptitude rather than one of inaptitude in our work with the elderly? In fact, knowing that cognitive losses increase with age, practitioners must stay alert but continue to act without condemning every older adult at first sight (Browdie, 1993; Mixson, 1995; Anetzberger et al., 1997; Landau, 1998; Simmons & O'Brien, 1999).

In cases where older persons are completely capable and autonomous, practitioners presuppose that they are able to give informed consent to a particular proposal, and, therefore, their refusal of certain services is more easily accepted. This does not mean that their refusal must lead to a complete cessation in services offered (Gilbert, 1986; Matlaw & Mayer, 1988; Landau, 1988; Asch, 1993; Dresser, 1993; Browdie, 1993; Heisler & Quinn, 1995; Holstein, 1995; Anetzberger et al., 1997; Spencer, 1998; Simmons & O'Brien, 1999). On the contrary, there is meaning in investing in such a relationship. Perhaps older persons do not see a reason for services at a certain point in time, but with time, they will be better informed and feel more comfortable asking for help.

When the older adult is clearly incapable, a declaration of inaptitude can be requested as well as the establishment of protective supervision (advisor, tutorship or curatorship to persons of full age). These cases generally pose less problems for psychosocial practitioners working in the public system or in community organizations in view of the fact that elders are then taken in charge by specialised proceedings. Once again, authors emphasize the importance of minimal intrusion in the life of older persons (Mixson, 1995; Thomas, 1997; Marin et al., 1995; Heisler, 1995).

Situations that generate the most doubt and awkwardness for practitioners are cases where they question the older person's capacity to come to a decision. In fact, this occurs in cases where the person has partial aptitude. It seems that this is common in interventions with mistreated older adults; moreover, we may wonder if this partial aptitude is not a direct consequence of the abuse. Therefore, a close follow-up and periodical evaluations of psychological and physical capacities are necessary. Yet, practitioners cannot lose view of the fact that an incapability to verbally communicate is not equivalent to an incapability to decide (Matlaw & Mayer, 1986; Kane, 1993; Dresser, 1993; Asch, 1993; Marin et al., 1995; Heisler, 1995; Mixson, 1995; Sonntag, 1995; Heisler & Quinn, 1995; Spencer, 1998; Landau, 1998; Bergeron, 1999)!

(3) Confidentiality versus Collaboration Between Practitioners and Agencies

Effective actions pertaining to mistreatment rest on the collaboration and cooperation between practitioners and agencies (Spencer, 1998; Bergeron, 2001; Wolf & Pillemer, 1988). The sharing of information between professionals is crucial, given that interventions in situations of mistreatment can hardly be undertaken by a sole practitioner. Confidentiality constitutes a current dilemma in case management, particularly in situations that require the collaboration of practitioners of the same organization or of several different organizations. We enquire: in what cases do we need the consent of the client to communicate information (Kane et al., 1993)? The evaluation of the risk, as well as the restriction on the disclosure of information, is of paramount importance. Inversely, as emphasized by Spencer (1998), the principle of confidentiality, which is not absolute in any professional code, should not serve to legitimate inaction. Furthermore, we recognize ethical viewpoints as shifting, conditional on the profession and/or service. It is important to bear in mind that the ethical practice is composed of listening, searching for compromises fastened in the client's history, and adopting a vision that goes beyond the client's refusal. Some difficulties result from a lack of time and non-existent resources for proper follow-ups (Johnson, 1995; Holstein, 1995; Marin et al.,

1995). Health, public security, and social services organizations, which as a rule collaborate together, can offer a tighter safety net to abused older adults. It is important to prioritize collaboration in order to avoid authority interventions, which place simultaneously the client and services at risk. Mediation could be a solution, yet it is not always appropriate (Spencer, 1998).

(4) Social or Family Responsibilities?

Intervening with mistreated older adults introduces itself in a range of conditions, from social responses to social problems. Yet, concretely, who holds responsibility for the dependent elderly: families or the state? (Spencer, 1998). If families are responsible, what means are they given? If the state is responsible, why are we not more critical regarding health and social services offered to the elderly? What margin of action do practitioners have in their own organization? How can they exercise their professional autonomy and express their clinical judgement? (Beaulieu & Giasson, 2005). In order to be considered within their organization, shouldn't practitioners serve simultaneously the needs of the client and those of the system? The absence of resources, as well as the lack of time to devote to each case, permits practitioners to pass responsibility to each other. This creates tensions for everyone, including the abused older adult, who is oriented in several directions (Matlaw & Mayer, 1986; Browdie, 1993; Spencer, 1998). The availability of resources constitutes a factor for intervention quality in addition to client well-being. Is there not reason to worry with regards to non-existent resources in organizations as well as employment of either barely or not trained professionals to specifically intervene in issues of older adult mistreatment? The lack of resources in home-care services encourages practitioners to resort to inappropriate or unsafe solutions (Sonntag, 1995). In keeping with Bergeron (1999) and Asch (1993), there is reason to wonder: what is the purpose of laws without sufficient resources?

As emphasized by Sonntag (1995), in several countries, the responsibility of services offered to dependent older persons is handed over to the families, which is first and foremost a moral circumstance rather than a legal one. When families give treatment and services, practitioners owe it to them to properly evaluate available resources in order to avoid caregiving becoming a burden (Kane et al., 1993; Asch, 1993; Dresser, 1993). What are the primary interests of family members when they solicit the state for services to help their elderly family member? Do they want, as Mixson (1995) points out, to assure safety for their kin rather than respect their autonomy? Or, do they wish to allow their older relative to continue to live autonomously by reducing constraints?

(5) The Balance Between Competing Values in Practice

Frequently, questions arising from the practice are tinted by an implicit ethical reflection, which challenge practitioners and force them to position their intervention more solidly. They cover all dimensions of action, starting from the moment the problem is recorded, transiting from the decision to act or not, to the impacts of actions or lack of actions in the life of all the implicated parties: victim, abuser, and practitioner. The first question concerns the importance of taking or not taking action. Let's keep in mind that detecting and reporting may counter autonomy. Practitioners must understand the reasons to detect and evaluate a particular situation ensuring that the victim's profile requires it. Due to limited services, we have to remember that detection without possible action leads to discouragement for everyone (Gilbert, 1986; Saveman, 1992; Landau, 1998; Spencer, 1998). In contexts where protection laws for mistreated older adults exist, is it likely that the consequences stemming from the declaration of the abuse be worse than the informal accountability assumed by others? Or, then again, that the declaration be inappropriate or useless (Gilbert, 1986; Matlaw & Mayer, 1986; Kane et al., 1993; Anetzberger et al., 1997; Landau, 1998). Prior to making a complaint, the practitioner should evaluate the situation and the risks by emphasizing the involvement of some kind of non-intrusive protection for the victim (Matlaw & Mayer, 1986; Willbach, 1989; Anetzberger et al., 1997; Spencer, 1998). If there are only suspicions of mistreatment, it is preferable to avoid advancing further in the detection and denouncing process, but rather, to continue to offer a pro-active support to the victim (Saveman et al., 1992; Spencer, 1998).

Concerning intervention with older adult victims, what is the most important? Their physical or socio-affective needs? (Asch, 1993; Dresser, 1993; Spencer, 1998). It is certainly important to evaluate to what extent our service system is able to protect the victim. Unfortunately, numerous errors can potentially produce harmful consequences for the elderly (Landau, 1998).

Despite the fact that less documentation exists, practitioners greatly question themselves as regards to their actions with people who abuse or neglect older persons. It is suggested that persons who mistreat be given the possibility of obtaining a follow-up with a practitioner not involved with the victim (Marin et al., 1995). In some cases, a clear message must be sent to aggressors regarding their responsibility for their actions, by means of justice and compensation (Heisler & Quinn, 1995; Spencer, 1998). In fact, only a handful of lawsuits pertaining to older adult mistreatment actually make it to court in Québec. We can only deplore the fact that little or nothing has been written on effective accompaniment programs for persons who mistreat older adults.

In a perspective of ethical reflection, we can only emphasize the importance given to practitioners' actions or lack of actions. Ethical judgement is required to unmistakably identify the violent act or negligent behaviour in order to prevent confusion or neutrality from surfacing (Willbach, 1989; Saveman et al., 1996; Spencer, 1998). Beneficence, without consideration for the autonomy of older persons, can lead them to feel distressed even when their mental functions are reduced (Simmons & O'Brien, 1999).

Finally, in a context where several researchers are pleading for the development of clearer policies and better specified laws in the matter of mistreatment, it is important to remember that our theoretical models which allow us to understand and explain older adult mistreatment are still at the early babbling stages. Prudence is in order in light of the fact that our elaborated theories, stemming from incomplete knowledge, lead to inappropriate laws and practices (Bergeron, 2001).

METHODOLOGY

The value of research, after all,
depends not on some platonic measure of worth
but on its value for appropriate audience.
(Strauss, 1987, p. 301)

(1) Data Collection

The data analyzed come from a study pertaining to ethical issues of psychosocial intervention in situations of elder abuse.[3,4] The collection of data was conducted by using a qualitative approach. As Gubrium and Holstein say, we are part of the group of those "qualitative researchers interested in the social accomplishment of meaning and order" (2000, p. 487). Recruitment took place in two regions in Québec, Canada. The sample is composed of sixteen practitioners, eight from Québec City (4 from the community sector, 4 from the public sector) and eight from the Bas-Saint-Laurent (same disposition).[5]

For the purpose of the study, we retained two selection criteria: participants have worked for at least five years as psychosocial practitioners with an elderly clientele and possess significant intervention experience in situations of older adult mistreatment. Participants were recruited by means of the snowball technique, and we did not meet any practitioners from the same organization. We interviewed fourteen women and two men, with a work experience ranging from five years to approximately thirty years.

Practitioners were asked to describe their professional practice experiences in relation to their interventions with a clientele of abused older adults and their abusers. It was the same research professional, using a semi-structured approach, who conducted each interview. The interview protocol was divided in four sections: (1) perceptions concerning older adults in general and abused older adults in particular; (2) a description surrounding interventions (examples included problems, issues, and personal experiences); (3) a depiction of the rapport between intervention and society (examples included own values, and establishment of beliefs); and (4) a clarification of personal incentive for the chosen field and other personal questions. Practitioners were asked to express themselves with regards to their practice by using actual cases. This approach facilitated the emergence of ethical dilemmas. Data from interview transcripts were analyzed using N'Vivo, according to the mixed approach by Huberman and Miles (1991); that is, by combining inductive and thematic analysis.

For validation purposes, each practitioner received a written verbatim copy of his interview and was given the opportunity to comment on it, even to "correct" it, or minimally nuance it, prior to the analysis. The primary researcher and a group of research assistants carried out the thematic analysis performed according to the mixed approach (Huberman & Miles, 1991).

For the purpose of this article, we translated several quotes from the original French data. It gives a sense of the richness of our material.

(2) The Approach by Principle in Ethical Intervention Research

The approach by principle was originally developed by bioethics, a discipline created to respond to issues and scientific developments as well as technical dilemmas in the health services field. At the outset, it was applied to clinical intervention and research; now it is starting to be used in the public and community health sectors. In this respect, our project is original. Beauchamp and Childress (1979, 2001) in *Principles of Biomedical Ethics*, present a method, which consists of a reflection as well as the resolution of ethical dilemmas, structured around four principles: respect of autonomy, beneficence, non-malfeasance, and justice. In this approach, values are not in competition with one another; rather they complement each other. As a result, the decision to act in one way or another reflects a balance between values.

As illustrated in Figure 1, each value is not only theoretical, it is also transformed and adapted in order to guide the application. In our analysis, we account for these values. Even though we had introduced specific questions on ethical issues of the practice, we rapidly realized that the practitioners were much more comfortable naming ethical reflections and dilemmas in an implicit manner.

RESULTS AND DISCUSSION

One of the key issues in social work in the future
may be how professionals work with clients in this area
to acknowledge their individuality and adulthood
when there is public pressure to protect and pity.
(Manthorpe, 1994, p. 88)

(1) Psychosocial Intervention

Intervention in situations of mistreatment of older adults can be described on a practice continuum. On one end of the continuum, we find negative autonomy, and at the other end, extreme measures, and finally, in the centre, accompaniment measures (see Figure 2). The choice of one type of practice over another depends on the evolution of three variables: the loss of autonomy of the older person, the dangerousness of the situation and the collaboration between the three parties (victim, abuser, and practitioner). These conditions can vary slowly or rapidly (an increasing dementia or a stroke; the departure of a caregiver; an increased number of violent or neglectful events). Changes or deterioration in any one of these variables influence the intervention process in place. Therefore, there is room for questioning the fragility of the clinical relationship.

Negative autonomy occurs when a person refuses the proposals of the practitioner. The latter chooses to withdraw from the file and accepts the refusal of the client. Intervention then comes to an end. It is abandonment of the victim rather than concrete intervention.

Accompaniment is the ideal condition. Decisions are made in a gradual fashion depending on the case and the relationship between the practitioner

FIGURE 1. Bioethical Principles as Applied to Intervention

Values	Application
Respect of the person's autonomy	Establish conditions for a decisional process that respects the person's autonomy
Beneficence/non-malfeasance	Minimise disadvantages and maximise benefits in relation to intervention goals
Justice	Respond to needs without discrimination and with impartiality

FIGURE 2. The Intervention Process

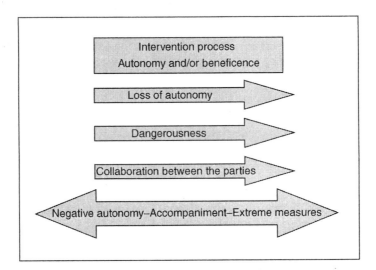

and the client, and occasionally, the relationship between the practitioner and the abuser.

Extreme measures are taken when practitioners are forced to make important decisions in a short period of time. These decisions are sometimes made without either the absolute consent of the older adult victim nor the complete collaboration of the abuser.

In their remarks, practitioners consider themselves quite preoccupied by the respect of autonomy of older persons and are concerned by their protection (therefore, beneficence) rather than non-malfeasance or justice. In fact, it appears that these two previous values are relegated to second and third place. The following quote illustrates this balance between values and the type of feelings generated in practitioners:

> What is important, my priority, it is the respect of the client, what he wants to do. But, it is not evident though. What he wants to do and what he should do, are two things. We can never decide for them unless they are really in danger for themselves or for others, that the person be dangerous for herself or for others and those that live with her never realize to what point . . . like someone with Alzheimer's that would not realize that she is really subjected to mistreatments. Therefore, we have a great deal of worry because we do not have much power to intervene, when the person says no, we get going again, we are empty-handed but we are

conscious of the danger, we are conscious of the probability of death. But my greatest fear is to find myself with someone who gets killed.

(2) Values at Play in Psychosocial Intervention

I think that one of the values is respect with regards to the person, and once we have that respect for the person, it will inspire all interventions we may have . . .

What emerges from participants' accounts is respect as a meta-value that transcends all actions. This respect of the person guides the construction of values that stimulate the practice, whether it is negative autonomy, accompaniment or extreme measures.

When the refusal of services by victims is entirely respected without any attempt to pursue the intervention, it is considered negative autonomy. With the hopes of not influencing the victim in their choice, the practitioner is exiting a situation that contains a certain level of risk, which may degenerate over time. This practice of abandonment or the lack of recognition of mistreatment raises some questions, as mentioned by a practitioner:

In fact, what I want to say is that with regards to statistics it is practically at 10% . . . It is not normal that there are practitioners that never make any statistical references. It is not possible that in their caseload of sixty, seventy files, that they do not have situations of abuse. Sometimes I tell myself, is it because they do not work with them or that they do not dare see them, they don't touch that, or, they work with them but they don't tell me. In any case, I think there are certain people that are more sensitive to that.

On the other hand, rather than completely respecting the person's autonomy, the practitioner is sometimes required to resort to extreme measures. The older adult in this instance is no longer fully autonomous and, therefore, is unable to care for him/herself and is incapable of defending his or her interests. The practitioner is caught between doing what is right for the older adult victim (beneficence) and preventing any harm to be experienced (malfeasance) by remaining vigilant with regards to the person's autonomy. This protection issue is often presented as a solution of last resort.

When all the strategies, intervention plans that we can imagine of which I was making reference to earlier (were tried), and we arrive in extreme situations where there is in fact a person who is abused, mistreated, who risks her life sometimes or whose capabilities are lessened and we tell ourselves, now, the only possibility, for example, is a home for the elderly. Ultimately, we must move towards protective supervision.

In accompaniment, the practitioner will ascertain that the person's autonomy is respected and remain vigilant regarding beneficence. Therefore, autonomy will be favoured but the practitioner will also encourage the victim to become active in the situation. He will continue to monitor the situation and will suggest some actions that are more focused on protecting the victim, but only when those actions are necessary.

As we have seen in the literature review pertaining to the pre-construction and axiological framework, practitioners are aware that their experience, their knowledge of ageing, as well as their own values, tint intervention. The following quote is an example of it:

> I began working at 22-years-old at the CLSC, I had a caseload of 90 elderly persons . . . I don't know if I said it, but I surely thought that I was working for the elderly . . . That changed a lot and my desire to want to change (the clientele) for every year in the beginning, maybe the first 5, 6 years, I was not comfortable with the older clientele. We worked with death, illness, so that's it. I had chosen a profession where we are in the problems, that's for sure, except I was not comfortable. The palliative care, the elderly, Alzheimer, tinkle, pooh, I did not always feel like talking about that. It's confronting, we see ourselves growing old, I was 22-years-old, so, no . . . it took me a long time to become comfortable. I would say that it has not been that long, because I had the opportunity to change clientele and I didn't do it. Therefore, it shows that now I am comfortable with that clientele, very comfortable. But, at a young age, 22-years-old, we do not have first-hand experience, and we do not have the same vision of the elderly also.

(3) The Psychosocial Practice

> We have to, of course, when it is necessary, protect them as much as possible. But not baby them, especially. They are ageing adults and they also have a part of responsibility with regards to their life. That, for me, is quite important. But, it is certain that in situations where there is an illness settling in, it is certain that they are more vulnerable and they need other people, that for me is clear.

In their practice, when practitioners wish to completely respect the older adult victim's refusal of services, they will close the file. Henceforth, there will not be any type of follow-up in the case. This is negative autonomy, and there are no practical interventions!

In cases of accompaniment, practitioners will prefer to intervene in a proactive manner. They will remain vigilant with regards to the situation that poses a risk. As a result, a number of these risks can be managed and certain crises anticipated. Consequently, the practitioner is able to generate unique protection scenarios adapted to the situation of the victim. The greatest challenge is creating a durable relationship, maintaining contact, and, most importantly, developing a relationship of confidence with the mistreated older adult. Victims are encouraged to take certain actions (empowerment), are given suggestions to compensate for their changing level of autonomy, and are accompanied in the distancing process between themselves and the situation of violence. Throughout this development, the victim gains greater self-knowledge. As well, the intention of the practitioner is to preserve or improve the victim's quality of life (such as respecting life habits, values, and culture) as well as enhance and extend his/her social support network, which also includes working with the victim's abuser. Practitioners act as advocates for the victim's rights, and their role is to influence, convince, modify beliefs, raise awareness, and so on. They call upon community organizations for partnership and are supported by interdisciplinary teams. The following situation illustrates an accompaniment in progress:

> Little by little, we created this connection with this women . . . at some point, after a certain amount of time, after creating a bond, well, I opened up to this women, about worries that I had in relation to risk, in relation to the presence of that man. Clearly we do not arrive in the first interview with that . . . People don't want to change things. The idea is to remain available, namely we say: "Listen, I respect that, that you do not want to, but if ever you change your mind, I am always there." The idea is not to close the door.

Finally, when practitioners resort to extreme measures, they are faced with some degree of urgency. They must protect the victim to the best of their knowledge, respect their mandate, and apply, when necessary, protective supervision. There are certain legal recourses that the practitioner can suggest to either the victim or his/her family, which they can choose, such as: divorce, protective supervision, Curator, court order (the only measure to force long-term care), accompaniment with legal procedures, assistance to lodge a complaint, and so on. In the event of great danger, poor collaboration on the part of the family as well as severe loss in the autonomy of the victim, the practitioner must resort to the removal of the older adult victim from the environment.

As we noticed in the literature review, practice is highly conditioned by the older person's capability, which seems to be treated in two ways: (1) comprehension or autonomy of the victim in relation to what is happening, and (2) the recourse of applying a legal disposition when the person finds him/herself in a high risk situation as well as incapable. For practitioners, the worst situation is when a person is under evaluation for protective supervision. Due to long delays, the person continues to live in a situation of risk whereas no one can adequately assure her safety.

(4) Issues Raised in Psychosocial Intervention (Figure 3)

4.1 Negative Autonomy

Relating to negative autonomy, the practitioner ceases to intervene in an elder abuse case when the client refuses any further services. The practitioner is comfortable with this situation when the person is autonomous, has the neces-

FIGURE 3. Issues Raised in Psychosocial Intervention

Negative Autonomy	Accompaniment	Extreme measures
–Comfortable when person is autonomous, capacity, informed decision (but uneasiness when there is resistance from the victim and doubts on his cognitive autonomy) –Result from: organization of services (voluntary context), lack of time, overwork, and the growing number of clients –Limited definition of autonomy –Powerlessness of the practitioner, resignation, withdrawal, denial = end of the intervention –Lack of training, awareness-raising, and supervision of the practitioners	–Obtain the person's consent –Time consuming intervention –Challenge = respect the person's rhythm –Constant evaluation process (autonomy, dangerousness, vulnerability, cognitive losses, etc.), –Requires vigilance, tools/scale/guidelines, and time –Live with an at-risk situation (tolerate certain risks that are lower than the negative consequences of a radical intervention). –Some discomfort related to the respect of autonomy (questioning of certain decisions made by the victim) –Equilibration process	–Maximal vulnerability of the victim –Crisis, hospitalization, or other change –Pressures in the agency (supervisor, colleagues,) –Pressures from the victim's entourage –Mandate, responsibility of the agency –Negative feelings (stressed, jammed, powerless, disappointment) –Professional autonomy level –Clinical support offered to the practitioner?
Abandonment of the older adult victim to himself	*Acceptance and tolerance of an unsafe situation*	*Continue to act with the older adults instead of for the older adult in a context of decision-making for the client and not by the client*

sary aptitude and makes an informed decision. However, uneasiness is felt when there is resistance from the older adult victim and there are doubts on his/her cognitive autonomy. This kind of situation causes some issues to be raised. When an older person victim resists services offered, should interventions be stopped? Certain questions arise: Does the older person completely understand the risks and consequences involved of this refusal? Are practitioners respecting the older person's autonomy when they choose to close the case instead of trying other forms of intervention? Practitioners are faced with a particular reality. They work in a voluntary context, which means they must respect the person's decisions and work around the fact that there are no legal measures to support actions that go beyond an older person's wishes in a case of violence other than when there is impending danger for the victim. More often than not, the practitioner is overworked (due to a disproportional ratio between the number of practitioners and the number of clients) and lacks the required time to accomplish all the necessary actions in a case of abuse and/or neglect. Intervention may come to a halt due to the practitioner's sense of powerlessness, which leads to relinquishment, withdrawal, and denial. Hence, a value conflict arises, for instance, by respecting a person's autonomy, are we acting in his/her best interest? Respecting a person's autonomy does not mean abandonment. Part of the responsibility of leaving the older person victim to fend for him/herself is due to the lack of any or sufficient training, awareness-raising, and proper supervision offered to practitioners faced with cases of elder abuse.

4.2 Accompaniment

These are extreme means where we really try to do everything and sometimes tolerate certain risks that we would rather not but that may be slighter than the intervention we could pose to protect the person.

Accompaniment is the ideal situation in which a practitioner and an older adult victim can discover themselves. In the event of mistreatment, the practitioner may not be comfortable with ceasing services on the sole basis that he/she must respect the victim's autonomy. In intervention, it is crucial, if not absolute, to obtain consent from the older adult victim. Hence, the practitioner is faced with the challenge of respecting the person's rhythm. To do so, he/she must be comfortable with small achievements, such as the place and time the practitioner is given by the older person as well as the few propositions the older person agrees to (as modest as they might be). In essence, it marks the beginning of a relationship between two beings that develops amidst respect, trust, tolerance, and commitment. This intervention approach requires vigilance and time because periodic evaluations must be performed in order to en-sure the autonomy of the person, evaluate the level of dangerousness of the situation as well as the person's vulnerability, and finally, assess the person's cognitive functions. Therefore, practitioners require adequate tools, evaluation scales, guidelines, and time in order to feel secure and supported in the deci-sion-making process. They must be able to work with an older person despite the fact that the situation in which they find themselves has risk potential. While several threats are out of the practitioners' control, they must exert tolerance in regards to certain risks that are lesser than the negative consequences of a radical intervention. The key qualities to possess in order to succeed in the accompani-ment measure are acceptance and tolerance in precarious situations.

4.3 Extreme Measures

> Wherever it is possible, I think we have to be very attentive at the outset, to just be aware. Is the act or the objective we are aiming for to reassure ourselves as interventionists or as a system, or is it really to bring more to the person who has a loss of autonomy?

Extreme measures are undertaken when the older adult victim experiences utmost vulnerability due, not only to the intensification of the mistreatment situation, but also to a dramatic change in the situation, for instance a crisis or a hospitalization. In such cases, practitioners are under extreme scrutiny. They are pressured by their colleagues to solve the situation as quickly as possible and by the victim's family members to have their wishes respected. Moreover, the message sent by society is one of accountability for intervening in a situation of mistreatment. In addition, practitioners must conform to their mandate and not overstep its boundaries. This tremendous amount of pressure may lead the prac-titioner to express negative feelings such as stress, powerlessness, disappoint-ment, and the sentiment of being in a dead-end. All these conditions may set the stage for ambiguous decision-making. Decisions must be made quickly, yet practitioners need to find themselves in favourable conditions in order to do so. Do practitioners have a sufficient level of professionalism as well as adequate clinical support to make such vital decisions?

We can see, from what practitioners have said, that there have been some changes in ways of working with older adults. These transformations stem from ethical reflections. In the past, practitioners were more often in extreme measures; today, they work in accompaniment. This change seems to be ex-plained by a better comprehension of their duties and powers:

Another ethical problem: It is certain that when you arrive in intervention, we have to use the real words when we talk about negligence also. We must say what we do, we have to inform. I would say: when we are confronted in working in a situation of incapacity, we owe it to ourselves to inform the person, even if we know we are moving towards a declaration of incapacity. Maybe previously we informed less and we did it, and we protected the person, and we determined that she was, between quotation marks, incapable. Yet, we do not have that role and we do not have that power. It is a court order that can determine the capacity of a person.

(5) Suggestions to Improve Intervention (see Figure 4)

I think there is a lack of training somewhere, the approach of violence against the elderly.

5.1 Negative Autonomy

Practitioners need to have adequate initial training in their field of study on the topic of violence and neglect. In the work place, ongoing training is necessary to consolidate acquired knowledge to what is asked in day-to-day practice. Furthermore, practitioners should be aware of the services offered in the community and adequately harmonize the client's needs to the appropriate services. Finally, practitioners have to receive support in the work place; they

FIGURE 4. Suggestions to Improve Intervention

Negative Autonomy	Accompaniment	Extreme measures
–Adequate initial and ongoing training –Resources in the community –Offer support to practitioners –Better application of the existing laws	–Clinical supervision –Possibilities for ethical discussions –Interdisciplinary teams –Collaboration between organizations –Provincial or federal framework to guide the practice	–Detection tools –A reinforced protective net –Possibilities to practice ethical decision-making (balancing the values of all parties)
–Offering proper detection tools in the identification of elder abuse	**–Guidance in clarifying cases of elder abuse and developing best practice**	**–Systematization of application procedures in cases of elder abuse and creation of an environment that pushes forward a meta-reflection on action**

need a place to verbalize their impressions of a situation as well as express how they feel. Therefore, it is essential that, if practitioners are to move beyond respecting autonomy, they should have good detection tools to facilitate the identification of elder abuse and neglect. As can be noticed in the following quote, the first steps often go unnoticed but remain fundamental:

> We especially try to raise the awareness of our work colleagues, all of the people that work with us: the nurses, the auxiliary workers. We make them aware, we do a lot of training, approaches to rapidly detect older adult abuse.

5.2 Accompaniment

At this stage, practitioners should have a good foundation derived from their initial training and the ongoing training as suggested in negative autonomy. Furthermore, sufficient clinical supervision on a regular basis ought to be prioritized as well as opportunities for discussions on ethical issues with the aim of helping practitioners perfect their practice. Better intervention competence suggests a greater synchronisation between needs and services. Practitioners find assistance and reinforcement in interdisciplinary team meetings as well as from collaboration between different organizations. Intervention could be improved by receiving greater support from the Provincial and Federal governments in guiding psychosocial practice by means of social policy.

In relation to the literature review, we observe that the question of collaboration between agencies not only raises issues about the level of accompaniment. In fact, there is reason to believe that economic and political imperatives can largely tint interventions, as the following citation reveals:

> So I think there are situations that are very litigious that we have to carry alone . . . I am thinking specifically of, when we make a request for a long-term care facility, or when we have a situation where the person is waiting for the opening of protective supervision with the Curator. As long as the court judgement is not made, the person is not declared incapable. Therefore, the Curator, it is not them that will go to court to obtain the long-term care facility request, it is the CLSC. So who will pay for the lawyer's fees? It is the CLSC. When we know that the person will be declared incapable, that the file is already sent to the Curator. There are financial and political issues.

The discourses of practitioners who find themselves in a situation of accompaniment are at times quite eloquent with regards to the distress not only of the victims but also of the abusers. They do not minimize the fact that some persons who mistreat the elderly are dangerous or malicious people, but they also present the opposite side of the coin by proposing a reflection on social responsibilities that we have towards families. In this way, the following quote illustrates the reflection proposed in the literature review on the topic of family and social responsibilities in relation to mistreatment of older adults. What should be done when the informal carer is burdened?

> She had said to the practitioners of the CLSC: Me, I am so tired, I don't know how long I will last. And she had said: I am afraid of myself to some degree. That is why a social practitioner would go to her home. Because, starting from the moment where people say: "I am afraid of me," it means: "I don't know how I can react."

5.3 Extreme Measures

When practitioners are faced with cases of extreme vulnerability, they not only require clinical support, interdisciplinary assistance, collaboration with other organizations and adequate social policies, but also require proper clinical tools that take into consideration all of these aspects. Good collaboration with the victim's family is crucial in order to facilitate any necessary changes for the older adult victim. In the decision-making process, as time-consuming as it might be, the values of everyone ought to be considered and decisions should include all parties involved. When advancing towards extreme measures in cases of elder abuse, systematization is required in order to apply procedures effectively.

Many of the recommendations presented above point towards greater training development and adapted work tools. It does not consist necessarily of rigid protocols or procedures but rather of the production of material and adapted practical guides. As we have mentioned previously, few practitioners received the appropriate training on the topic of mistreatment of older adults. Questions are raised as a result of gaps in the practice. Certain practitioners even wonder why it is so difficult to transfer training experience from conjugal violence to mistreatment towards the elderly.

> In matters of conjugal violence, we must meet the person . . . The conjugal therapy on abuse-violence-neglect . . . we believe a lot more in individual intervention. But if there is a will, if the notion of abuse is settled and there is a willingness towards a conjugal therapy, well, of course it will be more . . . In fact, it is what we tell one person and what we tell another, and the importance that if we suspect that there is abuse, if the couple wishes to have a follow-up in conjugal therapy, well, it is clear that it will not be the same practitioner that discovered the abuse. I think that on

this we have to question ourselves sometimes. In fact, we often say in conjugal intervention, it is rare that we will go for conjugal therapy in a situation of abuse-violence-neglect. But there has been conjugal therapy anyway after an abuse, we cannot hide that.

CONCLUSION

I would say that, in general, what bothers me a little with regards to violence, money laundering, is really really bad ! But to beat an elderly person, that is less bad!

Whether it is in theory or in practice, issues related to intervention in situations of mistreatment of the elderly trigger many psychosocial and ethical questions. It is evident from the verbatim that one can not simply classify practitioners as being more or less in favour of autonomy or as being instantly in favour of protective supervision for the elderly. Of course, some practitioners deplore the fact that some of their colleges do not see anything or practice a form of negative autonomy, but the 16 practitioners interviewed showed a great deal of openness and discernment. In fact, the practice depends on numerous objective and subjective factors, the most important being the older person's loss of autonomy, the dangerousness of the situation and the collaboration between parties (victim and abuser). It is possible for a case to move through the entire continuum. In the beginning, it may not be detected or followed-up (negative autonomy), then it may become added to a regular caseload (accompaniment), and lastly, it may require one or more directive interventions (extreme measures).

The results from our study allow us to validate among practice history and practitioners' reflections with regards to their work, the collection of psychosocial issues and identification of ethics in the literature review. The original dimension of our work was to give central actors, the practitioners, full opportunity to speak. To our knowledge, we are also the first to propose a practice continuum inspired by an ethical reflection concerning action by identifying values in the practice: promoting the equilibrium between autonomy and beneficence/non-malfeasance. Furthermore, we are surprised to notice that practitioners do not speak about justice. In our opinion, justice should be more readily considered as a value if only to denounce moral vices or flaws in the application of legal procedures (particularly, protective supervision) or better yet, condemn the fact that other types of crime, such as money laundering, are more severely punished than mistreatment towards the elderly. Would it not be interesting to understand this modest preoccupation for equity?

Problems revealed by the practice are numerous and practitioners do not conceal their malaise, their worries, and even their incompetence or their limited power to intervene in certain cases. The reflection that arose from this study in order to expand and improve the practice, as rich and innovative as it is, does not permit us to be quite as affirmative as are Brownell and Wolden (2002), in their comparison of benefits and limits in social work centered approaches as well as criminal justice approaches, to effectively respond to different forms of violence and neglect.

Our work leads us to many research avenues. We now better know the ethical and psychosocial issues encountered by psychosocial practitioners when working with mistreated older adults in the community. What type of challenges are facing psychosocial practitioners working in emergency rooms, in nursing homes or long-term care settings? What are the challenges for other practitioners such as nurses, psychologists, and physicians? How could validated detection or intervention protocols influence the issues raised by the practice? As well, it would be interesting to perform a case study over several months in order to capture and understand the ethical and psychosocial dilemmas of all actors who are part of the situation (mistreated older adult, the abuser, other family members or people of trust, social worker, nurse, and physician). This would allow us to better understand the evolution of intervention and its impacts.

Many of the findings of this study could be transformed into useful training material. We must not only prepare our future practitioners to work with cases of mistreatment of older adults, but also train and support the practitioners in all agencies that work directly or indirectly with mistreated older adults. Other than what the rich content suggests such as, what mistreatment entails, how it is recognized, how to intervene with the victim, how to work with the abuser, what legal and social possibilities exist in offering support, and so on, we have to be prepared to teach practitioners how to develop the capacity to intervene in grey areas and in evolving situations that hold a high risk potential. Practitioners need to know and share their concerns facing the fact that there is never a precise answer to the question: "How far do we go?" We also have a certain amount of responsibility in encouraging all agencies to introduce some ethical dimensions to case discussions. It is worth pursuing ethical reflection; in other words: let's dialogue.

NOTES

1. This disposition says that "every aged person has a right to protection against any form of exploitation. Exploitation means taking advantage of the vulnerability or dependency of an elderly person to deprive that person of his or her rights, for example, by extorting money, inflicting abuse, withholding care that is required for health,

safety, or well-being, or attacking the person's dignity" (Commission des droits de la personne et de la jeunesse, 1975, p. 7). It is important to acknowledge that this disposition has been in force since the mid '70s but less than 10 cases were completely processed. It is then a very unusual solution to mistreatment of older adults.

2. These two studies were conducted by telephone with older adults living in the community. It excludes all the institutionalized adults, those with hearing problems or without telephone. More so, the main methodological limit to these studies is their incapacity to control the presence or not of the abuser nearby the older adult during the interview.

3. This research was funded by the Social Science Research Council of Canada, Grant: 410-2000-1541.

4. The P.I., Marie Beaulieu, wishes to recognize the contribution of Ghyslaine Lalande, Annie Lévesque, Josée Roy, Josée Mainville, Francine Caron, Mylène Giasson, and Nancy Leclerc at different stages of the 4 years project.

5. This project has received an ethical approval from the University of Québec in Rimouski and the University of Sherbrooke. All practitioners also signed a written consent form prior to the data collection.

6. The Figures 2 to 4 are a translation and adaptation of an initial figure published by Giasson and Beaulieu (2004). The authors wish to acknowledge the contribution of Milène Giasson at the results section.

REFERENCES

Anetzberger, G. J., Dayton, C., & McMonagle, P. (1997). A community dialogue series on ethics and elder abuse: Guidelines for decision-making. *Journal of Elder Abuse & Neglect, 9* (1), 33-50.

Asch, A. (1993). Abused or neglected clients–Or abusive or neglectful service systems? In R. A. Kane & A. L. Caplan (Eds.), *Ethical Conflicts in the Management of Home Care.* (pp. 113-121). New York: Springer Publishing Company.

Beauchamp, T. L., & Childress, J. F. (2001). *Principles of Biomedical Ethics.* New York: Oxford University Press.

Beaulieu, M. (1992). Elder abuse: Levels of scientific knowledge in Québec. *Journal of Elder Abuse & Neglect, 4* (1/2), 135-149.

Beaulieu, M., Gordon, R., & Spencer, C. (2003). *An Environmental Scan of Abuse and Neglect of Older Adults in Later Life in Canada: What's Working and Why.* Research report prepared for the Federal, Provincial, and Territories Ministers responsible for Seniors, p. 69

Beaulieu, M., & Giasson, M. (2005). *L'éthique et l'exercice de l'autonomie professionnelle des intervenants psychosociaux œuvrant auprès de personnes aînées maltraitées. Nouvelles Pratiques Sociales 18*(1), 131-147.

Bergeron, L. R. (1999). Decision-making and adult protective services workers: Identifying critical factors. *Journal of Elder Abuse & Neglect, 10* (3/4), 87-113.

Bergeron, L. R. (2001). An elder abuse case study: Caregiver stress or domestic violence? You decide. *Journal of Gerontological Social Work, 34* (4), 47-63.

Bergeron, L. R., & Gray, B. (2003). Ethical dilemmas of reporting suspected elder abuse. *Social Work, 48* (1), 96-105.

Bookin, D., & Dunkle, R. E. (1985). Elder abuse: Issues for the practitioner. *Social Casework: The Journal of Contemporary Social Work, 66* (1), 3-12.

Browdie, R. (1993). View from the field: Perspective from Pennsylvania. In R. A. Kane & A. L. Caplan (Eds.), *Ethical Conflicts in the Management of Home Care* (pp. 128-129) New York: Springer Publishing Company.

Brownell, P., & Wolden, A. (2002). Elder abuse intervention strategies: Social service or criminal justice? *Journal of Gerontological Social Work, 40* (1/2), 83-100.

Commission des droits de la personne et de la jeunesse. (1975) *The Québec Charter of Human Rights and Freedoms.* (R.S.Q.C.-12). *http://www.cdpdj.qc.ca/en/home.asp? noeud1=0&noeud2=0&cle=0*

Dresser, R. (1993). Values and perspectives on abuse: Unspoken influences on ethical reasoning. In R. A. Kane & A. L. Caplan (Eds.), *Ethical Conflicts in the Management of Home Care* (pp. 121-127). New York: Springer Publishing Company.

Fulmer, T. (1991). Elder mistreatment: Progress in community detection and intervention. *Family and Community Health, 14* (2), 26-34.

Fulmer, T., & Peveza, G. (1998). Neglect of the elderly patient. *Nursing Clinics of North America, 33* (3), 457-466.

Fulmer, T., Guadagno, L., Pavesa, G. J., VandeWeerd, C., Baglioni, A. J., & Abramson, I. (2002). Profiles of elder adults who screen positive for neglect during emergency department visit. *Journal of Elder Abuse & Neglect, 14* (2), 26-34.

Giasson, M., & Beaulieu, M. (2004). Le respect de l'autonomie: Un enjeu éthique dans l'intervention psychosociale auprès des aînés maltraités. *Intervention, 120,* 98-109.

Gilbert, D. A. (1986). The ethics of mandatory elder abuse reporting statutes. *Advances in Nursing Science, 8* (2), 51-62.

Gubrium, J. F., & Holstein, J. A. (2000). Analyzing Interpretative Practice. In N. K. Denzin & Y. S. Lincoln (Eds.), *Handbook of Qualitative Research* (2 ed.) (pp. 487-508). Newbury Park: Sage Publications.

Heisler, C. J., & Quinn, M. J. (1995). Legal perspective. *Journal of Elder Abuse & Neglect, 7* (2/3), 131-156.

Holstein, M. (1995). Multidisciplinary ethical decision-making: Uniting differing professional perspectives. *Journal of Elder Abuse & Neglect, 7* (2/3), 169-182.

Huberman, A. M., & Miles, B. M. (1991). *Analyse des données qualitatives. Recueil de nouvelles méthodes.* Bruxelles: De Boeck.

Johnson, T. F. (1995). Ethics and elder mistreatment: Uniting protocol with practice. *Journal of Elder Abuse & Neglect, 7* (2/3), 1-18.

Kane, R. A., Penrod, J. D., & Kivnik, H. Q. (1993). Ethics and case management: Preliminary results of an empirical study. In R. A. Kane & A. L. Caplan (Eds.), *Ethical Conflicts in the Management of Home Care* (pp. 7-25). New York: Springer Publishing Company.

Landau, R. (1998). Ethical dilemmas in treating cases of abuse of older people in the family. *International Journal of Law, Policy & the Family, 12* (3), 345-355.

Manthorpe, J. (1994). Elder Abuse and Key Areas in Social Work. In P. Decalmer & F. Glendenning (Eds.), *The Mistreatment of Elderly People* (pp. 88-101). London: Sage Publications.

Marin, R. S., Booth, B. K., Lidz, C. W., Morycz, R. K., & Wettstein, R. M. (1995). Mental health perspective. *Journal of Elder Abuse & Neglect, 7* (2/3), 49-68.

Matlaw, J.-R., & Mayer, J.-B. (1986). Elder abuse: Ethical and practical dilemmas for social work. *Health and Social Work, 11* (2), 85-94.

Mixson, P. M. (1995). An adult protective services perspective. *Journal of Elder Abuse & Neglect, 7* (2/3), 69-87.

Podnieks, E., Pillemer, K., Nicholson, J. P., Shillington, T., & Frizzel, A. (1990). *National Survey on Abuse of the Elderly in Canada.* Toronto: Ryerson Polytechnical Institute.

Pottie Bunge, V. (2000). Mauvais traitements infligés aux adultes plus âgés par les membres de la famille. In Statistique Canada (Ed.), *La violence familiale: Un profil statistique* (pp. 29-33). Ottawa: Centre canadien de la statistique juridique.

Randal, J., & German, T. (1999). *The aging and development report: Poverty, independence, and the world's people. London, Help Age international.* www.who.int/entity/violence_ injury_prevention/violence/global_campaign/en/chap5.pdf.

Saveman, B.-I., Norberg, A., & Hallberg, I. R. (1992). The problems of dealing with abuse and neglect of the elderly: Interviews with District nurses. *Qualitative Health Research, 2* (30), 302-317.

Saveman, B.-I., Hallberg, I. R., & Norberg, A. (1996). Narratives by District Nurses about elder abuse within families. *Clinical Nursing Research, 5* (2), 220-236.

Simmons, P. D., & O'Brien, J. G. (1999). Ethics and aging: Confronting abuse and self-neglect. *Journal of Elder Abuse & Neglect, 11* (2), 34-54.

Sonntag, J. (1995). Case manager's perspective. *Journal of Elder Abuse & Neglect, 7* (2/3), 115-130.

Spencer, C. (1998). Ethical dilemmas in dealing with abuse and neglect of older adults. *Ethica, 10* (1), 71-74.

Strauss, A. (1987). *Qualitative Analysis for Social Scientists.* Cambridge: Cambridge University Press.

Thomas, N. D. (1997). Hoarding: Eccentricity or pathology: When to intervene? *Journal of Gerontological Social Work, 29* (1), 45-55.

Villani, P. J. (1994). *Ethics and Values in Long-term Care.* Binghamton, NY: The Haworth Press, Inc.

Willbach, D. (1989). Ethics and family therapy: The case management of family violence. *Journal of Marital & Family Therapy, 15* (1), 43-52.

Wolf, R. S., & Pillemer, K. A. (1994). What's new in elder abuse programming? Four bright ideas. *The Gerontologist, 34* (1), 126-129.

World Health Organisation (2002). The Toronto Declaration on the Global Prevention of Elder Abuse, *http://www.who.int/hpr/ageing/TorontoDeclarationEnglish.pdf*

Elder Abuse and Neglect Among Veterans in Greater Los Angeles: Prevalence, Types, and Intervention Outcomes

Ailee Moon, PhD
Kerianne Lawson, MSW, MSG
Maria Carpiac, MSW
Eleanor Spaziano, MSW

SUMMARY. This study examined the prevalence, types, and intervention outcomes of elder abuse/neglect among a veteran population. A review of medical records of 575 veterans who had received services from the Veteran's Affairs Geriatric Outpatient Clinic in Los Angeles during a three-year period found 31 veterans (5.4%) who had an elder abuse report filed on their behalf. Prevalence of elder abuse/neglect was higher among older (80+) and Caucasian and African American veterans. Eight of 31 victims suffered from more than one type of elder abuse including self-neglect. Financial abuse and self-neglect were the most commonly reported types. Family members were perpetrators in the majority of the cases, excluding self-neglect. However, three-quarters of financial abuse cases were committed by non-family members. Almost one-half of the victims had dementia and eight were clinically depressed. The most common intervention was to move victims from their unsafe home into a

[Haworth co-indexing entry note]: "Elder Abuse and Neglect Among Veterans in Greater Los Angeles: Prevalence, Types, and Intervention Outcomes." Moon, Ailee et al. Co-published simultaneously in *Journal of Gerontological Social Work* (The Haworth Press, Inc.) Vol. 46, No. 3/4, 2006, pp. 187-204; and: *Elder Abuse and Mistreatment: Policy, Practice, and Research* (ed: M. Joanna Mellor, and Patricia Brownell) The Haworth Press, Inc., 2006, pp. 187-204. Single or multiple copies of this article are available for a fee from The Haworth Document Delivery Service [1-800-HAWORTH, 9:00 a.m. - 5:00 p.m. (EST). E-mail address: docdelivery@haworthpress.com].

nursing home or board and care facility, followed by conservatorship arrangement. These interventions were most frequently used for victims with dementia, and conservatorship was often arranged with another type of intervention, such as a move to a nursing home. Victims who remained at home received conservatorship or outside supportive services or a combination of both. This study calls for more comprehensive and systematic research on elder abuse/neglect at multi-settings in order to generate useful information for prevention and detection of, and effective intervention in elder abuse and neglect in the veteran population. *[Article copies available for a fee from The Haworth Document Delivery Service: 1-800-HAWORTH. E-mail address: <docdelivery@haworthpress.com> Website: <http://www. HaworthPress.com> © 2006 by The Haworth Press, Inc. All rights reserved.]*

KEYWORDS. Elder abuse, veterans, prevalence, intervention outcomes

INTRODUCTION

Research on the prevalence of domestic elder abuse in the past two decades has reported different rates of prevalence, ranging from one to ten percent (Brownell & Abelman, 1998: Gioglio & Blakemore, 1983; Lau & Kosberg, 1999; National Center on Elder Abuse, 1998; Pillemer & Finkelhor, 1988; Swagerty et al., 1999; Young, 2000). The wide variations in these findings, to some extent, reflect major differences in the research methods employed by the studies, including sample size and sampling method, location and method of data collection, and operational definition and measurement of elder abuse and neglect. However, this earlier research has made a significant contribution to the illumination of the dark reality of a silent suffering of a vulnerable segment of the aging population in the United States, emphasizing the importance of recognizing elder abuse and neglect as a serious social problem. Indeed, elder abuse poses serious harm to the physical, psychological, financial, and social well-being of older people.

The problem of elder abuse is growing. A national study conducted by the National Center on Elder Abuse (NCEA, 1997) found that reported domestic elder abuse and neglect cases rose from 117,000 in 1986 to 293,000 in 1996, an alarming increase of 150 percent. Another study (NCEA, 1998) estimated that in 1996 approximately 450,000 elderly persons in domestic settings were abused and/or neglected. The study further revealed that only 16% of these cases were reported to and substantiated by Adult Protective Service (APS) agencies.

In California, the number of elder abuse and neglect cases reported to APS has been increasing at a fast rate: In September 1999, 3,654 cases were reported and the number rose to 5,487 in September 2003, or an increase of 50% in four years (California Department of Social Services, 1999, 2003). California state officials estimated that APS served only seven to nine percent of older adults at risk of being abused or neglected (California Department of Social Services, 2000). In addition, in a study of Non-Hispanic White and Korean immigrant elderly in Greater Los Angeles (Moon & Kim, in progress), 19% of White elders and 39% of Korean immigrant elders reported at least one incident of elder abuse or neglect that had occurred to their relative, friend, or neighbor in their own racial/ethnic circles during the past 12 months. These findings clearly suggest that elder abuse is a pervasive but hidden problem posing many challenges to policy makers, service providers, and researchers in search of effective elder abuse prevention, detection, and intervention.

Elder Abuse Victim and Perpetrator Characteristics

Research on elder abuse has also focused on identifying characteristics of victims and perpetrators, suggesting that a typical victim is over 75 years of age, a female, has debilitating physical and psychological impairments, and is dependent upon a family caregiver, usually a daughter (Falcioni, 1982; Hirst & Miller, 1986; Kosberg, 1988, 1998; O'Malley et al., 1983; Pillemer & Finkelhor, 1988; Ramsey-Klawsnik, 1991, 1993). For example, Kosberg (1988) identified the characteristics of elders at high risk of abuse as being female of advanced age, dependent upon others for care, problem drinkers, individuals with histories of intergenerational conflicts, those who internalize blame, display excessive loyalty towards caregivers, or who have suffered abuse in the past, and those who are isolated or impaired and display stoicism or provocative behavior.

While elder abuse is perpetrated by non-family members as well as by family members, research has consistently shown that the most common perpetrators of elder abuse are spouses and adult children (Chang & Moon, 1997; Moon & Kim, in progress; Pillemer & Finkelhor, 1988; Ramsey-Klawsnik, 1991). Kosberg (1988) also suggested that caregivers who are at high risk for inflicting elder abuse include substance abusers, those who suffer psychological impairment, are economically dependent, inexperienced in providing care to others, have a history of childhood abuse, are unengaged outside the home, display blaming or hypercritical behavior, lack understanding and sympathy, and have unrealistic expectations and stress.

Some studies have focused on identifying characteristics of victims and perpetrators by type of abuse (Coyne, 1991; Coyne et al., 1993; Dyer et al.,

2000; McDonald, 1996; NCEA, 1998; Pillemer & Suitor, 1992). For example, McDonald (1996) in a review of findings from major studies in this area indicated that older persons with dementia who exhibit disruptive behavior and live with family caregivers are at high-risk of physical abuse, and their abusive caregivers may suffer from low self-esteem and clinical depression (Coyne, 1991; Coyne et al., 1993; Pillemer & Suitor, 1992). Victims of financial abuse are usually unmarried or widowed, have relatively poor health, and are socially isolated, and victims of neglect tend to be very old with cognitive and physical impairment. Depressed older adults are more likely to experience neglect or self-neglect (Dyer et al., 2000), and self-neglect among those who abuse alcohol is common as they may neglect their health, and become depressed or isolated from their social network (Blondell, 1999). Wolf (1994) concluded that physical and psychological abuses are more closely associated with the problems of the perpetrators than the victim.

The NCEA's (1998) national study on domestic elder abuse reported that women were the victims in 60% to 76% (60% of self-neglect and 76% of emotional abuse) of the reported cases for each type of abuse, and individuals 80 years of age and older were the victims in 41% of reported emotional abuse cases and 52% of reported neglect cases. Only 23% of the reported victims in the study were fully able to care for themselves, and almost 60% were either very confused or somewhat confused. While approximately two-thirds of the victims were women, men were slightly more likely to be perpetrators, and 90% of the perpetrators were family members or relatives (47% child, 19% spouse, 9% grandchild, and 15% sibling or other relative). With the exception of the African American elderly population, ethnic minority elderly groups were under-represented among victims of all types of abuse and neglect: White and African American older adults accounted for over 96% (79.0% and 17.2%, respectively) of all substantiated elder abuse and neglect cases.

Elder Abuse in the Veteran Population

Despite growing research on elder abuse, little is known about the problem of elder abuse among the veteran population and of the unique role military service may play in the occurrence of elder abuse. In fact, veteran status has not been considered in previous studies of elder abuse. However, as Spiro and colleagues (1997) suggested, military status may affect the aging process of veterans, particularly for those exposed to combat, which may be partially responsible for physical and psychological health outcomes of elderly veterans. In addition, military service may affect some veterans' ability to form relationships and function in civilian society, thereby placing elderly veterans in a particularly vulnerable position for elder abuse and neglect victimization. The current cohort of elderly veterans is predominantly male. Men are more likely to be concentrated in vulnerable situations such as boarding homes, single occupancy hotels and prisons and are more likely to be homeless, users of alcohol or other substances, and in poor physical health than their female peers (Kosberg, 1998). This points to the importance of examining elder abuse and neglect in the veteran population.

The present study is a first step toward filling the gap in elder abuse research on the veteran population. Specifically, it describes the prevalence, types, perpetrators, and known intervention outcomes of elder abuse and neglect among veterans in Greater Los Angeles.

METHODS

Study Site, Source of Data, and Sample

The Geriatric Research, Education, and Clinical Center (GRECC)'s Outpatient Clinic of the West Los Angeles Veteran's Affairs (VA) Medical Center was chosen as a study site because of the accessibility to patient enrollment lists and documents about specialized geriatric services provided to the elderly veterans. The GRECC's Outpatient Clinic offers the expertise of an interdisciplinary team, consisting of instructional attending physicians, geriatric fellows, social workers, psychologists, psychiatrists, pharmacists, nutritionists, and medical interns and students. Elderly veterans are referred to the Clinic through the hospital's internal consult service for outpatients and inpatients. Veterans with a long history of multiple medical problems, poly-pharmacy issues, unique geriatric issues, or psychosocial needs are referred by the primary care provider who feels that the needs of the patient can be better served by the expertise of the GRECC's team and the availability of the GRECC social worker who also functions as a case manager.

This secondary data analysis examined anonymous retrospective data through medical chart review and social work assessment and referral form reviews in accordance with the guidelines required by the Veteran's Affairs Institutional Review Board (VA IRB). Specifically, demographic information (age, gender, and race/ethnicity) used in this study was extracted from the VA's computer-based patient records system. The diagnosis of dementia and depression was taken from a Social Work Assessment and Referral Form completed by the GRECC social worker upon initial assessment with each patient and was either self-reported or diagnosed by the GRECC interdisciplinary team. The Social Work Assessment and subsequent notes in the patient's file contain information about abuse and neglect suspected and reported to APS or to the police.

Due to limitations in the manner in which GRECC's patient rosters have been maintained, the rosters were available for 1998, 2001, and 2002, and data up to and including April 25, 2002 were used for analysis. Patient rosters were compiled and duplicate names were stricken from the lists. This resulted in a final sample total of 575 GRECC patients.

Identification and Analysis of Elder Abuse Cases

The Social Work Assessment and Referral Form and subsequent notes were reviewed for indications of abuse or neglect reported to Adult Protective Services (APS), in accordance with the Welfare and Institutions Code of California, which mandates "any licensed staff of a public or private facility that provides care or services for elder or dependent adults" to report "known or suspected" abuse to the authorities (W&I § 15630). Indications of abuse or neglect were most commonly identified by a phrase such as "APS report filed today" with a detailed description of the nature and circumstance of the abuse, the perpetrator's relationship to the victim, physical and mental health conditions of the victim, safety issues, available resources, need for intervention services, and in subsequent notes, outcome of the GRECC social worker's intervention. According to the GRECC social worker, about one-half of the reported abuse or neglect cases were self-disclosed by the patients themselves.

Instances of abuse or neglect were then recorded as classified by the social worker as one or more of five types: physical, psychological, financial, neglect, and self-neglect. Physical abuse was defined as "the use of physical force that results in pain, impairment, or bodily injury" (Gray-Vickrey, 2001, p. 37). Physical abuse included slapping, punching, biting, pulling, burning, pushing, and the use of physical or chemical restraints. Psychological abuse was defined as "the willful infliction of anguish through threats, intimidation, humiliation, and isolation" (Ibid.). Financial abuse was defined as "the illegal or improper use of an elder's resources for profit or gain" (Blunt, 1996, p. 62), which included fraud, theft, misappropriation of funds, property, or assets, and extortion (Bond et al., 1999). Neglect was defined as the failure to provide food and water, withholding medication or medical attention, and withholding emotional support or attention. Self-neglect was defined as the failure to maintain personal care, shelter, and health care at acceptable levels (O'Brien et al., 1999).

The perpetrator of the abuse was recorded as categorized by the social worker as self, spouse, adult child, friend, partner (non-spouse), or other (including neighbors or unknown perpetrators) and could include multiple abusers. Location of the abuse was categorized dichotomously as either home or facility (such as a board and care or skilled nursing facility). Outcome of the GRECC social worker's intervention was recorded and categories were formed through a process of content analysis. Categories were: conservatorship, police report, institutionalization in a skilled nursing facility or board and care, home health care, psychotherapy, remaining at home, refusal of services, and unknown outcome. Diagnoses of dementia and depression were recorded as dichotomous variables ("yes" indicated the presence of dementia or depression and "no" indicated the absence of respective illness).

For all 575 elderly veterans 65 or older who had received services from the GRECC, including 31 victims of elder abuse or neglect, information on the gender, age, and ethnicity was recorded. For every elder abuse or neglect case, the type of abuse, relationship of the perpetrator to the victim, presence of dementia and depression in the victim, and intervention outcome were gathered.

FINDINGS

Demographic Characteristics of GRECC Patients and Elder Abuse Victims

Table 1 depicts the demographic characteristics of the GRECC's total patients served during the three-year period and those who were reported to APS as suspected elder abuse or neglect cases. It shows that of 575 GRECC patients, 31 veterans, or 5.4%, were reported to APS for further investigation and intervention.

Comparison of the characteristics of the APS-reported elderly veterans with those of the total GRECC roster suggests that the prevalence rate of elder abuse or neglect is higher among female, older (80 or older) and Caucasian and African American veterans than among male, younger (under 80) and Asian Pacific Islander or Hispanic veterans. Most elderly veterans in the sample were male (96%) as they accounted for 94%, or 29 of 31 APS reported cases, at the elder abuse/neglect prevalence rate of 5.0% among male elderly veterans. Conversely, the two female veterans reported to APS made up a higher prevalence rate of 8.7% among the total 23 GRECC female patients.

APS-reported veterans ranged in age from 70- to 97-years-old, while the age range of the total sample was from 65 to 103 years. As shown in the Table, incidents of elder abuse/neglect were more prevalent among older veterans: None of the 34 GRECC patients under 70 years of age was found to be a victim of elder abuse/neglect, while the percentage of the GRECC patients reported to APS consistently rose from 4.0% for the 70-79 age group to 6.7% for the 80-89 age group, and then to 8.7% for the oldest group of age 90 or older. To

TABLE 1. Demographic Characteristics of GRECC Patients and Elder Abuse Victims

Characteristics	GRECC Patients (A) (N = 575)		APS Reports (B) (N = 31)		APS Reports as % of Total Patients
	f	%	f	%	[(B) ÷ (A)] × 100
Total	**575**	**100%**	**31**	**100%**	**5.4%**
Sex					
Male	552	96%	29	94%	5.0%
Female	23	4%	2	6%	8.7%
Age					
65-69	34	6%	0	0%	0.0%
70-79	227	39%	9	29%	4.0%
80-89	268	47%	18	58%	6.7%
90-103	46	8%	4	13%	8.7%
Race/Ethnicity					
Caucasian	261	45%	18	58%	6.9%
African Am.	155	27%	11	36%	7.1%
Asian/Pacific Islan.	79	14%	1	3%	1.3%
Hispanic	18	3%	1	3%	5.6%
Native American	1	0.2%	0	0%	0.0%
Unknown	61	11%	0	0%	0.0%

put it differently, the veterans who were 80 or older comprised 71% of all APS reported cases in this sample, while they accounted for 55% of the total GRECC patients.

Table 1 also shows that Caucasian and African American veterans accounted for 58% and 36% of all APS reported victims, respectively, while they made up 45% and 27% of the total GRECC roster. In contrast, only one Asian Pacific Islander (Filipino American) veteran was identified as a victim of elder abuse/neglect, representing 3% of the total victims, although Asian Pacific Islanders veterans constituted 14% of the total GRECC patients. Similarly, one of 18 Hispanic veterans seen by the GRECC was reported as a victim of elder abuse/neglect. As a result, the elder abuse/neglect prevalence rate was substantially higher for Caucasians (6.9%), and for African Americans (7.1%) than the average of 5.4% for the total sample and that of 1.3% for Asian Pacific Islander elderly veterans.

It must be noted that with the exception of one case, all of the reported elder abuse/neglect cases occurred in the community at the veteran's private residence. One case of neglect occurred at a nursing home where the veteran was residing at the time of the reported neglect.

Types of Abuse, Perpetrators, and Presence of Depression and Dementia

Table 2 presents findings on the types of abuse, perpetrators' relationships to victims, and the presence of depression and dementia in the victims. It shows that a total of 41 incidents or situations of elder abuse/neglect were identified among 31 victims: Eight victims (26%) suffered from more than one type of elder abuse, including self-neglect. Financial abuse and self-neglect were the most frequently reported types of abuse/neglect with 12 incidents each: They each represented 29% of the total incidents and affected 39% of the victims.

Examples of financial abuse were found in cases in which friends, neighbors, or family members gained control of and drained the veteran's bank account or situations in which power of attorney had been sought or granted when the veteran lacked decisional capacity. Self-neglect cases included el-

TABLE 2. Types of Abuse, Perpetrator's Relationship to Victim, and Presence of Symptom of Depression and Dementia in Victim (N = 31)

	frequency	percentage	
Type of abuse/neglect (n = 41)		% of n(41)	% of N(31)
Financial	12	29%	39%
Self-neglect	12	29	39
Neglect	7	17	23
Physical	5	12	16
Psychological	5	12	16
Perpetrator's relationship to victim (n = 37)		% of n(37)	% of N(31)
Self	12	32%	39%
Son	5	14	16
Spouse	5	14	16
Girlfriend/friend	5	14	16
Daughter	3	8	10
Neighbor	3	8	10
Niece	1	3	3
Homeless people	1	3	3
Unknown	2	5	6
Depression in victim			
Yes	11	NA	35%
No	20	NA	65%
Dementia in victim			
Yes	15	NA	48%
No	16	NA	52%

NA: not applicable

derly veterans living in unsanitary conditions and cluttered homes as well as some veterans who were suffering from dehydration or malnutrition.

Neglect was reported in seven cases, representing 17% of the total incidents affecting 23% of the victims. Neglect occurred most commonly due to the failure of family caregivers to provide needed personal care to the elderly veteran which often resulted in the development of a medical crisis that finally brought the needs of the veteran to the VA's attention. For example, a male elderly veteran with dementia was left alone for a week while his adult daughter, his primary caregiver, went out of town without arranging for anyone to assist him while she was gone: As a result, the veteran was hospitalized because he became hypertensive due to forgetting to take his medications.

Physical abuse occurred to five veterans. An example of this type of abuse occurred to an elderly wheelchair-bound veteran with numerous bruises, burns, and scabs on his legs and arms, who was abused by his grandson. The grandson shoved and yelled at him because he refused to give him money to buy drugs. An additional five veterans were abused psychologically or emotionally, such as a wife's insulting and angry comments about the elderly veteran's incontinence, a wife breaking the voice box machine of a veteran so that he could not communicate with anyone outside the home, and frequent threats of physical violence. No sexual abuse was found in this study.

As some cases involved multiple types of abuse/neglect, Table 2 also indicates that at least four cases, excluding the two unknown cases, involved more than one perpetrator. Considering the high percentage of self-neglect cases, it is not surprising that the victim himself or herself was the most frequent perpetrator with 12 cases, accounting for 32% of the total 37 perpetrators involved, or 39% of the total 31 cases. The remaining 25 perpetrators included spouses (5), son/stepson (5), friend or girlfriend (5), daughter (3), neighbor (3), niece (1), homeless person (1), and two unknown perpetrators. Excluding the victim for self-neglect and unknown perpetrators, family members (spouse, daughter, and son/stepson) made up 61% of the perpetrators.

Of the 31 victims of abuse/neglect identified in this study, 35% were diagnosed as clinically depressed, measured by the Geriatric Depression Scale (Yesavage et al., 1983). Almost one-half of the victims (48%) were found to be demented, measured by the Mini Mental Status Examination (Folstein et al., 1975), at the time of APS reporting.

As presented in Table 3, a closer examination of the 31 cases of elder abuse/neglect categorized by the perpetrator's relationship to the victim reveals several patterns. First, the findings indicate that the victim's wife was a perpetrator in at least half of the eight cases involving multiple types of abuse and also in four of the five physical abuse cases. Second, except for one case, family members, specifically spouse, son and daughter, were identified as per-

TABLE 3. Intervention Outcomes of Elder Abuse/Neglect Cases by Types of Abuse/Neglect, Perpetrator, and Diagnosis of Depression and Dementia (N = 31)

Type of abuse/neglect	Perpetrator	Depression	Dementia	Intervention outcome
Self neglect (10)*	Self (10)	Yes (2)/No (0) Yes (0)/No (2) Yes (2)/No (0) Yes (1)/No (3)	Yes (2)/No (0) Yes (2)/No (0) No (2)/Yes (0) Yes (2)/No (2)	C & NH (2) NH, C, & Home Health Care RS/Home (2) Unknown (4)
Financial (7)	Daughter/friend Friend (3) Neighbor (2) Niece	Yes Yes (1)/No (2) Yes (1)/No (1) No	No Yes (2)/No (1) Yes (1)/No (1) No	Police report Police report, C, C, & NH C, C, & BC RS/Home
Neglect (4)	Daughter Wife/son Son/daughter Unknown	No No No Yes	Yes No No Yes	NH Home w/home health care BC C
Psychological (2)	Son (2)	Yes (2)	No (2)	RS/Home Unknown
Neglect & financial (2)	Homeless person Unknown	No No	Yes Yes	C NH
Physical & self-neglect (1)	Wife & self	Yes	No	Home w/counseling
Physical & psych. (1)	Wife & stepson	No	No	Unknown
Physical & financial (1)	Girlfriend	No	Yes	C & NH
Financial & self-neglect (1)	Neighbor & self	No	No	RS/Home
Physical, psych., & neglect (1)	Wife	No	No	BC
Physical, psych., & financial (1)	Wife	No	No	NH

*The figure in the parentheses is the number of cases.
Note: C = Conservatorship; NH = Nursing home; RS/Home = Victim refused services and remained at home; BC = Board and care, including assisted living facilities; Unknown = Intervention or outcome was unknown to the VA because victims could not be located or they no longer contacted or returned to the VA.

197

petrators in all cases of neglect. This finding reflects the social norm that immediate family members ought to care for their elderly parents or spouse and the failure to do so is considered neglect. Third, three-quarters of the financial abuse cases were committed by non-family members: Nine of 12 identified perpetrators were friends (4), neighbors (3), girlfriend (1), and a homeless person (1).

Findings on the depression status of victims by type of abuse in Table 3 suggest that victims with depression were found in almost all types of abuse/neglect. In the absence of depression data on the general GRECC patient roster, however, it is difficult to assess the relationship between depression status and the prevalence of elder abuse/neglect. It is also possible that depression in elder abuse victims was a risk factor for some, but for others, it was a consequence of abuse. Nevertheless, the fact remains that over one-third of the victims were depressed. Table 3 also clearly suggests that dementia is a high risk factor for self-neglect, and to a lesser extent, neglect. For example, 7 of the 10 victims in cases of self-neglect only were veterans with dementia.

Intervention Outcomes of Elder Abuse/Neglect Cases

After an abuse/neglect case had been identified and reported to APS, the GRECC social worker further assessed the situation, paying particular attention to any threats to the victim's safety and health, as well as available resources and service needs, and then developed an intervention plan in consultation with the GRECC interdisciplinary team and/or APS. Table 3 presents intervention outcomes by type of abuse/neglect, relationship of the perpetrator to the victim, and diagnosis of depression and dementia.

Not all victims were willing to accept intervention services. In fact, five of 31 victims refused to receive recommended intervention services and remained at home ("RS/Home"). In addition, after APS reports had been filed, six victims never contacted the GRECC or returned to the VA system; nor was the GRECC able to locate them, making it impossible to provide intervention services. Consequently, these cases were classified as "unknown" for their intervention services or outcomes. As a result, 20 of the 31 victims (65%) were assisted with intervention services by the GRECC.

Table 3 further indicates that all seven cases involving neglect, including three cases of neglect occurring with other types of abuse, received service interventions, such as conservatorship, home health care, or moving into a nursing or board and care facility. It also shows that the most common intervention was to move 11 victims from their unsafe home into a nursing home (8) or board and care facility (3), such as an assisted living facility. For one victim of neglect, who was already living in a nursing home and who was diagnosed as being depressed and demented, a conservatorship was arranged on his behalf to prevent further neglect of his care needs at the facility. It is notable that moving into a nursing home or board and care facility was the most common intervention outcome for the victims with dementia: Among 20 victims with known and accepted intervention outcomes, 11 victims with dementia were living at their home at the time of abuse or neglect and seven of them moved into a nursing home or board and care facility.

Arrangement of a conservatorship was the second most common intervention, provided to ten victims. Conservatorship was also the most frequently used intervention for the victims with dementia, or those lacking decisional capacity and for financial abuse victims: Of the ten cases with a conservatorship as an intervention outcome, nine victims had dementia and six cases involved financial abuse. In addition, for six of the ten cases, conservatorship was arranged in combination with another type of intervention, including moving the victim into a nursing or board and care facility or home health care.

Of the 20 victims with known interventions, seven remained at their home and were provided either conservatorship or outside supportive services (home health care or counseling) or a combination of both. Finally, for two cases of financial abuse, whose perpetrators were a friend in one case and a daughter and a friend in the other case, were immediately reported to the police, and the outcomes of the police report were unknown.

DISCUSSION AND IMPLICATIONS

Before discussing the study's findings and their implications, it must be recognized that patients at one VA geriatric outpatient clinic are, by no means, a representative sample of the entire elderly veteran population. As mentioned earlier, patients were referred to the clinic for their geriatric, medical, and/or psychological service needs, and thus the sample most likely underrepresented healthy elderly veterans. This skewed sample, combined with its relatively small size for an elder abuse prevalence study, poses a major limitation to the generalizability of the study findings, which, therefore, must be interpreted with caution. Equally important to note is that the study findings, which were based on the information in the Social Work Assessment and Referral forms completed by the GRECC social worker, may reflect the social worker's biases, unknown to the researchers, in detecting and categorizing types of elder abuse or neglect, in assessing needs of veterans, and in planning for intervention. However, this bias is inherent in the role of the mandated reporter, who only has to have a suspicion of abuse to be required to report the situation to APS.

Despite these potential limitations, this exploratory study offers useful insight into the problem of elder abuse among elderly veterans. Most obviously, it clearly indicates that the elderly veteran is not immune to the problem of elder abuse and neglect: Among 575 elderly veterans, 31 victims of abuse and neglect, including self-neglect, or 5.4% of the total, was identified. Nineteen or almost two-thirds of the victims were abused or neglected by others. Considering the 1997 National Center on Elder Abuse (NCEA) study's finding that victims and heath care providers (hospitals, clinics, physicians, and nurses) consisted of only 35% of reporters of substantiated abuse by others, it is highly plausible that the elder abuse prevalence among the GRECC patients would be higher if such reports filed by other reporters, including family members, friends, neighbors, and in-home or out-of-home service providers outside the VA could be identified and included in the study.

In addition, the number of elder abuse and neglect victims could have been higher to the extent to which the social worker had failed to detect possible signs of abuse or neglect and patients had not disclosed potentially abusive or neglectful situations to the social worker for various reasons, including shame, guilt, self-blame, dementia, depression, and fear of retaliation by perpetrators. In fact, studies have suggested that some elder abuse/neglect victims may not tell anyone at all about abuse (Moon & Williams, 1993; Podnieks, 1992) and that many victims do not seek help from formal sources of help such as the police, APS, and social and health service providers, especially when the perpetrators are their children (Brownell, Berman & Salamone, 1999; Moon & Evans-Campbell, 1999; Moon & Williams, 1993; Phillips et al., 2000). Furthermore, some victims may view abuse as normal behavior (Phillips et al., 2000), and some victims may blame themselves for the abusive situation (Moon & Benton, 2000; Moon, Tomita, & Kamei, 2001; Podnieks, 1992; Sanchez, 1999). Indeed, detection of elder abuse and neglect poses a serious challenge to social and health service providers, and those working with the veteran population are no exception.

Compared to the NCEA's findings (1998) which found neglect as the most prevalent type of abuse (49%), followed by emotional abuse (35%) and physical abuse (26%), the current study's findings are similar with respect to neglect, including self-neglect, being one of the two most prevalent types of abuse and neglect (39%), although the percentage is lower than the NCEA's finding. In contrast, financial abuse among the veterans in the study was higher than in the national findings (39% versus 30%), and emotional/psychological abuse was significantly lower (16% versus 35%). For each veteran who presents for treatment at the VA, his or her Social Security and VA Disability income benefits are verified. This enables the GRECC social worker to detect major discrepancies between the verified amount of income from these sources and the amount reported by the veteran or veteran's family. This automatic income verification system at the VA seems to serve as a useful tool for detecting potential financial abuse. Lower rates of emotional abuse identified among the veterans may in part reflect the unique hospital setting as a study site and limited contacts veterans have with the health care providers or the GRECC social worker, which make it difficult to detect emotional abuse taking place in life situations outside the VA hospital or GRECC setting.

Focusing on the interventions, 20 veterans, or 65% of the total 31 victims, received intervention services. Unlike the situation in child abuse, elder abuse victims have the right to refuse services. Thus, one can argue that the percentage was not particularly low. A study of 401 cases of elder abuse in New York, for example, found that 70% of victims accepted services (Brownell et al., 1999). Nevertheless, the findings that 35% of the veteran victims did not receive any intervention service from the GRECC, including the six who could not be located nor were there records of whether or not they received needed services elsewhere, raise a serious concern about the safety and well-being of those victims. In this regard, there appears to be a serious gap in the collaboration and coordination between the VA and APS for intervention planning, service delivery, and follow-up to eliminate abuse/neglect and to assure the safety and well-being of the victims. This suggests an urgent need to institute an effective system of communication and coordination among APS, other legal authorities in charge of handling elder abuse and neglect, and social and health service providers.

It is also notable that none of the intervention arrangements seemed to have addressed the needs of the perpetrators, such as counseling, drug addiction treatment, and anger management. There is a growing consensus among researchers and practitioners that for some elder abuse victims, their desire to stop abuse and/or willingness to receive intervention services would be greater if they were ensured that the perpetrators would also be assisted with their problems and needs (Brownell, Berman, & Salamone, 1999). Evidently, all five cases of abuse and neglect inflicted by others for which the potential victims refused services, did not return to the GRECC, or the social worker was unable to locate the victims, involved family members as perpetrators (Table 3). Therefore, although it may go beyond the duty of the GRECC social worker at the VA hospital to assist non-veteran perpetrators, these research findings call for the inclusion of treatment plans for the perpetrators of the problem, which are vital for effective intervention aiming to stop elder abuse and neglect.

Finally, this exploratory study is only a first, small step in filling a gap in research and knowledge about the problem of elder abuse and neglect among elderly veterans. However, there is much to be done in future research. A comprehensive and systematic study of the prevalence of elder abuse and neglect in the general elderly veteran population is in order. In addition, a study of elderly veterans' perceptions of elder abuse, help-seeking behaviors, and knowledge of available services can provide useful information for addressing the needs of elderly veterans by developing effective public education programs to increase awareness of the problem, including risks and consequences, and available services, to enable early detection and intervention, thereby promoting safer and healthier lives of elderly veterans.

Future research should address social and health service providers' ability to detect elder abuse and neglect, their abuse assessment skills, and their intervention decisions. A lack of ability to detect, assess, and intervene in elder abuse and neglect results in the perpetuation or worsening of the suffering of elderly victims and inappropriate, ineffective intervention. Finally, on the systems level, research about weaknesses in collaboration and coordination efforts among social and health service providers, APS, the police, and other elder abuse related organizations, can provide useful insights for service and policy development for an effective societal intervention to stop the growing social problem of elder abuse and neglect.

REFERENCES

Blondell, R. (1999). Alcohol abuse and self-neglect in the elderly. *Journal of Elder Abuse & Neglect, 11*(2), 55-75.

Blunt, A. (1996). Financial exploitation: The best kept secret of elder abuse. *Aging, 367*, 62-65.

Bond, J., Cuddy, R., Dixon, G., Duncan, K., & Smith, D. (1999). The financial abuse of mentally incompetent older adults: A Canadian study. *Journal of Elder Abuse & Neglect, 11*(4), 23-38.

Brownell, P., & Abelman, I. (1998). Elder abuse: Protective and empowerment strategies for crisis intervention. In A. R. Roberts (Ed.), *Battered women and their families*. New York: Springer.

Brownell, P., Berman, J., & Salamone, A. (1999). Mental health and criminal justice issues among perpetrators of elder abuse. *Journal of Elder Abuse & Neglect, 11*(4), 81-94.

California Department of Social Services. (November 1999, 2003). *Adult Protective Services and County Services Block Grant Monthly Statistical Report*. Data Systems and Survey Design Bureau. *www.dss.cahwnet.gov/research/res/pdf/soc242*.

California Department of Social Services (May, 2000). *Early Impact of Senate Bill 2199: Opening the Door for Adult Protective Services*. Research and Development Division. Adult Programs Analysis Team.

Chang, J., & Moon, A. (1997). Korean American elderly's knowledge and perceptions of elder abuse: A qualitative analysis of cultural factors, *Journal of Multicultural Social Work, 6*(1/2), 139-154.

Coyne, A. (1991). The relationship between cognitive impairment and elder abuse. *Findings of Five Elder Abuse Studies.* Washington, DC: National Aging Resource Center on Elder Abuse, 3-20.

Coyne, A., Reichman, W., & Berbig, L. (1993). The relationship between dementia and elder abuse. *American Journal of Psychiatry, 150*(4), 643-646.

Dyer, C., Pavlik, V., Murphy, K., & Hyman, D. (2000). The high prevalence of depression and dementia in elder abuse or neglect. *Journal of the American Geriatrics Society, 48,* 205-208.

Dyer, C., Pavlik, V., Murphy, K., & Hyman, D. (2000). The high prevalence of depression and dementia in elder abuse or neglect. *Journal of the American Geriatrics Society, 48,* 205-208.

Falcioni, D. (1982). Assessing the abused elderly. *Journal of Gerontological Nursing, 8*(4), 208-212.

Folstein, M. F., Folstein, S. E., & McHugh, P. R. (1975). Mini-mental state. *Journal of Psychiatric Research, 12*(3), 189-198.

Gioglio, R., & Blackmore, T. (1983). *Elder abuse in New Jersey: The knowledge and experience of abuse among older New Jerseyans.* New Jersey: New Jersey Division of Youth and Family Services.

Gray-Vickrey, P. (2001). Protecting the older adult. *Nursing Management, 32*(10), 36-40.

Hirst, S. P., & Miller, J. (1986). The abused elderly. *Journal of Psycho-Social Nursing, 24,* 28-34.

Kosberg, J. I. (1988). Preventing elder abuse: Identification of high risk factors prior to placement decisions. *The Gerontologist, 28,* 43-50.

Kosberg, J. (1998). The abuse of elderly men. *Journal of Elder Abuse & Neglect, 9*(3), 69-86.

Lau, E., & Kosberg, J. (1979). Abuse of the elderly by informal care providers. *Aging, 297,* 10-15.

McDonald, L. (1996). Abuse and neglect of elders. In J. E. Birren (Ed.), *Encyclopedia of Gerontology: Age, aging, and the aged.* San Diego, CA: Academic Press.

Moon, A., & Benton, D. (2000). Tolerance of elder abuse and attitudes toward third-party intervention among African American, Korean American, and White elderly. *Journal of Multicultural Social Work, 8*(3/4), 283-303.

Moon, A., & Evans-Campbell, T. (1999). Awareness of formal and informal sources of help for victims of elder abuse among Korean American and Caucasian elders in Los Angeles. *Journal of Elder Abuse & Neglect, 11*(3), 1-23.

Moon, A., & Kim, S. (in progress). *Identification of elder abuse and neglect among Korean and White American Elderly.* Unpublished manuscript.

Moon, A., & Williams, O. J. (1993). Perceptions of elder abuse and help seeking patterns among African American, Caucasian American, and Korean American elderly women. *The Gerontologist, 33*(3), 386-395.

Moon, A., Tomita, S., & Jung-Kamei, S. (2001). Elder mistreatment among four Asian American groups: An exploratory study on tolerance, victim blaming, and attitudes toward third-party intervention. *Journal of Gerontological Social Work, 36*(1/2), 153-169.

National Center on Elder Abuse (1997). *Summaries of the statistical data on elder abuse in domestic settings for FY 1995 and FY 1996.* Washington, DC.

National Center on Elder Abuse. (1998). *The National Elder Abuse Incidence Study: Final report.* Washington, DC: National Center on Elder Abuse.

O'Malley, T., Everitt, D., O'Malley, H., & Campion, E. (1983). Identifying and preventing family medicated abuse and neglect of elderly persons. *Annals of Internal Medicine, 98,* 998-1004.

Phillips, L., Torres de Ardon, E., & Briones, G. (2000). Abuse of female caregivers by care recipients: Another form of elder abuse. *Journal of Elder Abuse & Neglect, 12*(3/4), 123-144.

Pillemer, K. A., & Finkelhor, D. (1988). The prevalence of elder abuse: A random sample survey. *The Gerontologist, 28*(1), 51-57.

Pillemer, K. A., & Suitor, J. J. (1992). Violence and violent feelings: What causes them among family caregivers. *Journal of Gerontology, 47,* S165-172.

Podnieks, E. (1992). National survey on abuse of the elderly in Canada. *Journal of Elder Abuse & Neglect, 4*(1/2), 5-58.

Ramsey-Klawsnik, H. (1991). Elder sexual abuse: Preliminary findings. *Journal of Elder Abuse & Neglect, 3*(3), 79-90.

Ramsey-Klawsnik, H. (1993). Recognizing and responding to elder maltreatment. *Pride Institute Journal of Long Term Home Health Care, 12*(3), 12-20.

Sanchez, Y. M. (1999). Elder mistreatment in Mexican American communities: The Nevada and Michigan experiences. In Tatara, T. (Ed.), *Understanding Elder Abuse in Minority Populations.* Philadelphia, PA: Brunner/Mazel, 67-77.

Spiro, A., Schnurr, P., & Aldwin, C. (1997). A life-span perspective on the effects of military service. *Journal of Geriatric Psychiatry, 30*(1), 91-128.

Swagerty, D., Takahashi, P., & Evans, J. (1999). Elder mistreatment. *American Family Physician, 59*(10), 2804-2811.

Wolf, R. S. (1994). Elder abuse: A family tragedy. *Ageing International,* March, 60-64.

Yesavage. J. A., Brink, T. L., Rose, T. A., Lum, O., Huang, V., Adey, M. B., & Leirer, V. O. (1983). Development and validation of a geriatric depression screening scale: A preliminary report. *Journal of Psychiatric Research, 17,* 37-49.

Young, M. (2000). Recognizing the signs of elder abuse. *Patient Care, 34*(20), 56-62.

Hearing the Voices of Abused Older Women

Jill Hightower, MA

M. J. (Greta) Smith

Henry C. Hightower, PhD

SUMMARY. This paper focuses on a qualitative research process that gathered responses from 64 older women aged fifty and older on their experience of violence and abuse. What older women said about abuse in their lives supports the use of a feminist framework as well as the age based analysis of the elder abuse field. Some respondents spoke of abuse from childhood into their later years. Some spoke of partners witnessing or experiencing abuse as children. Some women express concern about possible abuse by their adult children of their own children.

Abused older women like younger women need a safe environment, emotional support, advocacy, information, and peer support. While it is important to consider the perspectives and knowledge of service providers when developing policy and practice on abuse of older women, it is critical to ask the women survivors of abuse or neglect what they believe would benefit them, and others in similar situations. *[Article copies available for a fee from The Haworth Document Delivery Service: 1-800-HAWORTH. E-mail address: <docdelivery@haworthpress.com> Website: <http://www.HaworthPress.com> © 2006 by The Haworth Press, Inc. All rights reserved.]*

[Haworth co-indexing entry note]: "Hearing the Voices of Abused Older Women." Hightower, Jill, M. J. (Greta) Smith, and Henry C. Hightower. Co-published simultaneously in *Journal of Gerontological Social Work* (The Haworth Press, Inc.) Vol. 46, No. 3/4, 2006, pp. 205-227 ; and: *Elder Abuse and Mistreatment: Policy, Practice, and Research* (ed: M. Joanna Mellor, and Patricia Brownell) The Haworth Press, Inc., 2006, pp. 205-227. Single or multiple copies of this article are available for a fee from The Haworth Document Delivery Service [1-800-HAWORTH, 9:00 a.m. - 5:00 p.m. (EST). E-mail address: docdelivery@haworthpress.com].

KEYWORDS. Older women, domestic violence, elder abuse, ageism, feminist framework, Canada

In research policy and practice, when abuse of older women is addressed as a matter of elder abuse, the realities of the lives of women who are long term victims of abuse is missed. Age is not the major factor precipitating abuse of women in their fifties and older (Schaeffer, 1999; Morgan Disney & Associates, 2001; Hightower, 2001; Sargent & Mears, 2002; Scott & McKie, 2004).

This paper briefly discusses theoretical frameworks for research on older women. It then provides a summary account of an action-research project that examines the experiences of women of fifty and older in British Columbia, Canada who were victims of inter-personal violence and abuse. The methods used are primarily qualitative, community based, and informed by a theoretical framework using power and control and gender.

Older women shared with us stories of their abusive relationships with loved ones. Questions with obvious practice and policy implications were explored using this information. Why did they stay with their abusers? What help did they seek, and who helped or did not when asked? What changes would these women want, for others if not for themselves? How can outsiders comprehend violence within families?

Our premise is that while the current state of scientific theory prevails, it is essential to work with the women who have survived abuse or neglect if we are to develop effective policy and practice to address abuse in the lives of older women.

Individual women's stories in this research and similar research confirm and amplify two key lessons from the professional and academic literatures. First, domestic violence is often learned behaviour, and passed on from generation to generation. Second, it is all about power and control (Stewart, 2000; Anike, 1999; Kappel & Ramji, 1998; Schaffer, 1999; Sargent & Mears, 2000).

THEORETICAL FRAMEWORKS

Defining the Issue–Violence Against Women

The United Nations Declaration on the Elimination of Violence Against Women defines 'violence against women' to include

> Any act of gender-based violence that results in, or is likely to result in, physical, sexual, or psychological harm or suffering to women, includ-

ing threats of such acts, coercion, or arbitrary deprivation of liberty, whether occurring in public or private life. (United Nations, 1993)

Obviously, nothing in this statement excludes older women, or women of any age, from its scope. Others have noted a growing consensus that abuse of women and girls is best understood within a gender framework, since this abuse stems in part from women's and girls' subordinate status in society, and research and personal accounts of victims show that women's abuse by an intimate partner is generally a part of a pattern of abusive behavior and control (School of Public Health, Johns Hopkins University, 1999).

Women are the majority of the older population in virtually all nations (WHO/INPEA 2002, 3). In both the developing and developed world, older women are victims of poverty, inequality, and violence and abuse. While violence against women is recognized as a significant social, economic, and health problem, there is a general perception that it is a problem for younger women and that violent behavior within a family setting ceases with age. The reality is that women may experience abuse as children, at the hands of their parents, then by spouses or partners throughout their relationship, and in later years by their adult children (Hightower, 2004; Heise et al., 1994).

Defining the Issue: Elder Abuse

Elder abuse is defined as single or repeated act, or lack of appropriate action, occurring within a relationship where there is an expectation of trust, which causes harm or distress to an older person (Action on Elder Abuse, quoted by WHO/INPEA 2002). In addition to specifying age but not gender, this definition differs from a definition of violence against women in that the victim-perpetrator relationship is characterized as one of trust.

The image suggested by 'elder abuse' is of frail, dependent older people. Those who provide services for older adults are trained to understand the processes and complexities of aging and deal with age-related issues such as dementia and impaired mobility. For this reason, health providers are seen as well equipped to manage issues of violence toward older people (Sedger, 2001). Difficulties with this approach include its paternalistic and ageist implications. It ignores the criminality of acts that would be treated as criminal if the victim were of a younger age. This approach is exemplified in the development of services modeled on child protection, akin to a child abuse services model (Sacco, 1990; Vinton, 1997).

There has been much improvement with respect to violence in the lives of younger women where the common understanding of violence in intimate relationships has shifted, from seeing it as a private matter in which others have no right to intervene, to seeing it as a crime, which the state has an obligation to address. The 'elder abuse' label for violence in intimate relationships tends to leave crimes against older women, and they are crimes, still in the closet (Sedger, 2001). As noted in the *Missing Voices* report (WHO/INPEA, 2002), research in the field of Elder Abuse within a medical framework emphasizes pathology, and focuses on the characteristics of the perpetrator and the victim. There seems to be an underlying implication of "blaming the victim," particularly in research on caregiver stress.

These rationalizations seem to blame victims for being too needy and relieve perpetrators of responsibility for abusive action. In this age-based framework little attention is given to gender even though structures, interpersonal relations throughout the life cycle, and gender differences in aging reflect biological, economic and social differences that do not change in later years.

Whether the 'Elder Abuse' or 'Violence Against Women' framework is used when examining violence and abuse in the lives of older women, both approaches reflect a societal predisposition to homogenize older people by ignoring gender and individual differences. The result is that the needs of older abused women are not addressed. Given the reality of older women's lives our research framework involves a convergence of gender, and of age-related factors (Hightower et al., 2001).

FROM THE LITERATURE

The violence against women literature and the elder abuse literature have developed very separately and the theoretical differences are deep and difficult (Scott et al., 2003). Both have neglected the problems of violence against older women (Sargent & Mears, 2002). The realities of the lives of older women are lost when age alone is seen as a major factor precipitating abuse (Hightower, 2001). Older women's voices telling of their experience of violence are still rarely heard.

The ongoing violence and abuse in the lives of some older women gets little attention in the professional literature on violence against women. However, this is changing. Older women's advocacy groups and women serving agencies, particularly in Australia, Canada, United States, and Western Europe, have begun research, education and program development on this issue.

These groups do have some success in obtaining some government and foundation support for their work. However, unless they have access to the Internet and the financial resources to present their work at conferences, this community-based research, education and program development does not become part of professionally recognized knowledge. As in earlier years with domestic violence research, abuse of older women tends to be community driven, leaving academics and other professional researchers playing catch-up.

The gradual understanding that older women are still vulnerable to partner violence has resulted in some women's services developing specific programs for older women (NCEA, 1996). In Canada and the United States, advocacy activities have resulted in some cross training workshop materials being developed to bring together social and health services providers in the field of elder abuse with those providing services in the area of violence against women. Notable is the work of the Wisconsin Coalition Against Domestic Violence, Education Wife Assault in Ontario, and in British Columbia the BC Yukon Society of Transition Houses.

Medical journals such as *American Family Physician* are beginning to discuss screening older women for domestic violence (Mouton & Espino, 1999; Nudelman, 1999). Research on the impact of violence and abuse on women's health is growing and an article by Lachs et al. (1998) discusses the mortality of elder mistreatment. Our thesis on the gendered nature of continued violence and abuse in the lives of older women is supported by the medical findings of a recent national study of postmenopausal women in the USA (Mouton, Rodabough et al., 2004). A key finding of their research is that many functionally independent older women are exposed to physical and verbal abuse. "If a woman remains functionally independent, the risk factors for abuse mirror those for intimate partner violence" (Mouton et al., 2004, p. 609). Mouton and colleagues' summary conclusion is that "[older] women are exposed to abuse at similar rates to younger women; this abuse poses a serious threat to their health" (abstract).

Older Women's Voices as Reported in the Literature

An Australian women's health action research project in 1997 included the objective of identifying the needs of older women who are isolated and who were living or had lived in an intimate relationship with a violent partner. This project enabled older women to tell their stories and give their views on how to support their peers (Schaeffer, 1999:62). That phone-in study involved over 90 women between the ages of 50 and 78 who called to share their stories and give their ideas on what needs to be done to help other older women (Schaeffer, 1999:63).

This was followed by a national study on domestic violence in the lives of older men and women. The report documented the increased difficulty older women face in disclosing their abuse, which the authors attribute in part to socialization that included a widespread acceptance of violence (Morgan Disney et al., 2000).

The framework of Pritchard's report on the needs of older abused women in Britain (2000) is age-based, but the author highlights long term and complex needs of these older women. Of those she interviewed, 77% were women, and of those 64% were 75 or older. Most commonly the known abusers were male (66%), and physical abuse was involved in 58% of cases. What they needed to deal with the situations these women identified in their stories was very informed practical help, i.e., advice related to leaving abusive situations. They needed to know about places of safety, available housing, pensions and other benefits, personal financial issues, and obtaining a divorce.

"Older Women Speak Up" is the title of an Australian collection of life stories and vignettes by abused older women published in booklet form (Sargent & Mears, 2000). It was followed by a project report for older women in 2002 and a project report for professionals in 2002.

A research study on older women and domestic violence in Scotland (2004) mirrors the findings of the earlier studies. These researchers noted serious barriers older women face in accessing support, the lack of appropriate services. Barriers to service were said to be cultural and professional assumptions that older woman are not experiencing domestic violence, not believing the victim, traditional attitudes in later life about marriage and gender roles, exposure to long-term abuse, lack of independent income, and isolation from and lack of familiarity with the service system (Scott et al., 2004, p. iv).

Four projects in Canada at a community level that have focused on violence in the lives of older women are: A Study of Shelter Needs, prepared for the Older Women's Network in Ontario (Kappel & Ramji, 1998); Older Women Survivors: A Video and Handbook for and About Older Women who have Survived Abuse (*Older Women's Long-term Survival Society*, n.d.); and an analysis of the Impact of the Violence Against Women in Relationship Policy (VAWIR) on older abused women (Stewart, 2000). We include our ongoing work under the auspices of the B.C. and Yukon Society of Transition Houses as the fourth project, and will discuss it in more detail later. The themes echoed in interviews with survivors and documented in all these studies of older women's experience of violence and abuse in their earlier and present lives appear in our results, too. All this evidence seems to us to validate our conceptual framework of gender and age-related factors (Hightower et al., 2001).

METHODS

The primary data in this research project are limited to British Columbia. However, the use of physical and economic power for purposes of abuse and control is an essential element of child abuse, partner abuse, and abuse of older persons, and this crosses jurisdictional boundaries and is found in most if not all cultures. Thus the findings may be of use to people and agencies elsewhere.

A qualitative research process gathered responses from 64 older women aged 50 and older on their experience of violence and abuse. Older women who were being or had been abused at an older age were invited to tell their stories, describe their situations, and say what each thinks would help to keep her safe. In particular, the researchers wanted to know what services victims see as useful for themselves or others in their communities.

The design of this phase of the research borrowed much from work in Australia (Schaffer, 1999; Morgan Disney et al., 2000). The operational definition of 'older women' for this project included all women of age 50 or older. Any such criterion is necessarily open to attack for being arbitrary. From her experience with a survey in the United States that we replicated in a Survey of Women's Emergency Shelters in British Columbia, Dr. Linda Vinton recommended including women aged 50 to 60. This recognizes the particular financial difficulties faced by women who, because of limited prior work experience, and ageist attitudes, are unable to find employment above minimum wage levels, while they are still too young to access social security and old age pensions (Personal communication, 1998). Age 50 was also used in an Australian study (Morgan Disney et al., 2000) and a study on older women's needs in Ontario (Kappel & Ramji, 1998).

Data Sources

In cooperation with seven women's shelters and two multicultural immigrant support service agencies, a seven-day province-wide phone-in campaign was conducted. This replicated aspects of two projects in Australia (Schaffer, 1999; Morgan Disney et al., 2000). Through an advertising campaign, older women who were being abused or were survivors of family violence were encouraged to call toll-free numbers. The interviewers were counselors on the staffs of the shelters and cooperating agencies. This outreach activity was organized in conjunction with an annual public awareness campaign on the prevention of violence against women. A poster with a toll free phone number was produced and distributed to a broad spectrum of community services including women's shelters, women's resource centers, victim services agencies, community response networks, health centers, public libraries, and neighborhood houses, senior centers, and community heath centers. What is not really known is the number of posters that got displayed. Unfortunately, the publicity was affected by a sudden call for a provincial election and a major six-week transit strike in and around the Vancouver metropolitan area.

In addition to the phone-in, an invitation to contact us by mail was extended through the poster and in other ways. In some instances self-addressed, stamped envelopes were provided. The write-in campaign also used advertisements in local newspapers across the province inviting older women to mail their stories. This replicated an outreach project conducted in the United States by the American Association of Retired Persons (1996). Similar invitations, with additional contacts for information, were handed out at a seniors' conference, and to some Senior Citizen Counsellors. One of the researchers gave presentations on the project to a few seniors' groups and women's groups outside of metropolitan areas. Discussions with some Senior Citizen Counsellors and other service providers led to individual conversations with several older women survivors of abuse, and to a meeting with a group of older abused women. A gerontologist organized a similar meeting with another group of women. Data was also obtained from eleven individual interviews with older immigrant women, from a variety of foreign language groups, arranged through counsellors from their respective cultures. The interpretation and counselling skills of these counsellors were invaluable, as these older women could not have explained their situations in English to someone not familiar with traditions in their respective cultures of origin. Table 1 summarizes the sources of the data used.

Ethical Considerations

Interviewers who had volunteered in the seven women's shelters to answer the phones attended a briefing session to review the protocol and data collection sheets provided in an effort to get comparable baseline information from as many callers as possible. However, the primary point made in the protocol and briefing was that the first responsibility of the interviewer was to assess the current situation of the caller and ensure her safety. This reinforced the

TABLE 1. Sources of First-Person Data

Source	Women
Calls to the phone-in lines	15
Letters	16
Conversations after researcher's presentations	6
Group sessions (two groups)	16
Immigrant women interviewed with an interpreter/counsellor	11
Total	64

training and instincts of the shelter workers and counsellors who would be doing the interviewing. If the caller was currently living with or had recently separated from an abusive partner or children, she was asked if she was in a safe place when she made this call, if the police were involved, and if there were any weapons present. Depending on her answers, this might lead to on-line safety planning. She was asked if she wanted to leave the situation, and if she said she did at any time during the interview, she was offered a connection with a shelter in or near her community. Depending on the caller's response to this offer, she might no longer have absolute anonymity but would be promised confidentiality. This is counselling work, not interviewing. It was considered vital that people qualified as counsellors of abused women and well aware of the need to respect and maintain the anonymity or confidentiality of the caller answer these calls. Having first satisfied safety concerns, the data collection could proceed by asking the caller to tell her story, listening with encouragement as appropriate, and making notes on the key protocol items.

Anonymity was encouraged in invitations to write in, and stressed in phone conversations. Each woman in group meetings was given a one-page explanation of the project and assured of confidentiality. A counsellor who could assist and support the women was present at each of the group meetings and in the individual meetings with older immigrant women.

RESULTS

Assuming that some victims of domestic violence will be unwilling or unable to disclose their abuse, any survey that attempts to accurately measure the extent of a problem such as abuse of women by their loved ones is problematic. No attempt was made to estimate the proportion of older women who are abused. Instead, the focus was on providing information that would, it was hoped, inform those who by their administrative or legislative actions and professional services may make positive changes in the climate of opinion and provide services that raise awareness of opportunities for victims to change their lives and find safety and support.

The results are facts and conclusions are drawn from analysis of facts, but in general they are not quantitative facts and the analysis is not statistical.

Victims' Age

Some women interviewed by phone or who mailed in their stories said they were a First Nations person, or immigrant, or a woman with disabilities in the course of telling their stories. It is likely that other women in these and other visible or invisible minorities did not mention that, and minority status is not open to observation by phone or mail. The ages of the victims who mentioned their ages, as many did, ranged from 50 to 87 years, with 40% in their 60s and the average age being 67. Many of those who did not mention their age did provide other information that suggests an approximate age; for example, a woman who was married for fifty years must be close to if not into her seventies. We found no reason to think that any of those who did not give their ages were outside the 50- to 87-year-old range. The majority of their abusers were their husbands, though sons or daughters were the abusers of some of these women.

Nature of Abuse Suffered

We are not confident of the relative frequencies of types of abuse, alone or in various combinations, as we suspect there is a reporting bias with respect to types of abuse. Perhaps financial abuse is the easiest for an older women to articulate, and sexual abuse the most difficult to disclose, with physical and emotional abuse being somewhere in between those types. Even the term 'abuse' is somewhat taboo in this population, as some horrible acts, clearly criminal offenses, were described after victims began by saying something like, "I was not abused by my husband, perhaps just mistreated."

The women gave examples of physical, psychological, sexual, and financial abuse and violation of human rights. In more detail the variety of abuses that they had been subjected to by their husbands or, in some cases, their children involved psychological abuse in the form of harassment, verbal aggression, intimidation, insults, threats, and several kinds of enforced isolation. Monitoring and controlling outside contacts was also mentioned, often in combination with elements of financial abuse. Some of these cases involved withholding money for food and other basic essentials. Instances that involved financial abuse alone were generally associated more with sons or daughters rather than husbands. There were instances of sexual assault throughout married life. A few reports hinted at sexual abuse begun in later life but these remain ambiguous as it was difficult for the caller to share this information, and the interviewer did not want to probe into that area to minimize the real possibility of re-victimization through revisiting very painful experiences.

Duration of the Abuse

Some women told of life long abuse, from childhood in their family of origin, continuing through marriage, and sometimes re-marriage into another abusive relationship, and then into yet another. A woman who had been abused by her husband for almost all of their married life said:

> *I was brought up in a home with an alcoholic father and a 'rage-aholic' mother. During her rages she would often hit me on the head and swear at me. I thought seeing stars was a permanent condition.*

Some women disclosed that they had been in as many as three abusive relationships or marriages. For some respondents, as with some abused younger women, there is a pattern of moving in and out of the same abusive relationship a number of times.

There were only two instances in the data in which women with lifelong experience of abuse were still in abusive relationships. Again, it is suspected that selective non-disclosure may explain this result, as it is obviously easier, in both psychological and practical senses, to disclose abuse after it has ended than while living with the abuser.

Some of the women talked of their abuse continuing throughout their married life, until the death of their spouse. Several of those who had separated or divorced had been married, and abused, for twenty years or more.

Some older women were involved in a first abusive relationship started in later life. This happened after the death of a spouse, or in two cases, after they were divorced. As one woman explained, "I felt when I got married again that because I was 70 I wouldn't have these problems. It helps to know I can get help from people even though I'm older."

In some instances retirement seemed to increase the problems, as husbands became even more controlling. There was no mention in our data from older women of abuse connected to a husband's deteriorating health or related conditions.

Abuse by Adult Children

A small number of letters, phone calls, and interviews dealt with abuse by children. This abuse was nearly all financial and often involved housing and property.

This section of the paper has set out the basic information regarding the age, identity of the abusers, and length of the abuse. The following discussion expands on this information including their reasons for staying, what help they sought if any, who helped when asked, and what did they see as the needs of women like themselves?

DISCUSSION

Age and Abuse

As reported above, some of the women stated that their abuse had continued through their married life, until the death of their spouse. Several of the women who had separated or divorced had been married, and abused, for twenty years or more, and in one instance it was fifty years before she finally found the strength to get a divorce.

> *I was married 50 years until I divorced him five years ago. I had never lived alone. He was a rigid controlling man. It is good being on my own. Sometimes I feel so guilty for being so happy now.*

One woman over 80-years-old shared the story of her re-marriage in 1992. While she had some experience of abuse in a previous relationship, she said she had not spoken to anyone about the problem with her current husband, as she felt it was her responsibility to make the best of it, and she also felt ashamed. Her husband was very controlling, had a drinking problem, and always wanted money. Finally, she felt she just could not stand the confusion, verbal abuse, drinking, and girl friends any longer. She asked her family doctor for help. She was referred to a woman's shelter (transition house), and temporarily moved in with her son. She said that she was still feeling a little confused but found it very helpful to talk. She was now able to sleep at night and get some rest. She talked about selling her house and moving to another community where she thought she could get more help.

Retirement increased some difficulties, as husbands became even more controlling. Men who had had some authority in their work, it seems, transferred this aspect of their lives back into their homes. Among the things that the women mentioned were reorganization of kitchens, but obsessive control or nit picking over money was a very common concern in this context. There was one woman with health and mobility problems who said that as her husband got older, he became more cranky and had pushed and made her fall on several occasions. She remarked

> *I had a bad back, a degenerative spine disorder, and it became harder for me to get around. I needed my husband to drive me places more often. Sometimes he got cranky with me, or wouldn't take me. Anyway it got worse, and one time he pushed me and I hurt my hip.*

While there was no mention in our primary data of abuse connected to a husband's deteriorating health or related conditions, a contributor from Northern B.C., sharing the difficulties and needs of older women in more isolated areas, talked of the difficulty of an older woman being abused at the hands of a spouse who is developing a dementia and who has become aggressive and violent. It was pointed out to us that there are few services in rural areas for women in this situation. Another, perhaps even more difficult, situation shared with us was that of a woman who is herself developing dementia and is being abused by her "well" partner. If she is living in relative geographic isolation, she may rarely if ever see a service provider of any sort (Hemingway, 2001).

Abuse by Adult Children

The reported abuse by adult children was mainly financial and most often involved housing. One woman in her seventies talked of abuse from her daughter's boy friends. The abuse started about eight years ago, after her husband died. Several of her fifty-year-old daughter's boy friends have tried to get her to sign over her property. If she did not, they threatened; she would be alone and have no one. She did not do this, and she told them she is already alone. She has no further contact with her daughter and is seeing a counsellor once a month through the transition house. There were also stories of adult children encouraging their widowed mothers to sell their homes, to buy larger homes for themselves and the child and his or her partner, with disastrous consequences for the older parent. From what we heard from older women it would seem that estate planners should be cautious about encouraging older people to sign over their residences to their children for tax and estate benefits.

Life was often problematic for the older immigrant women interviewed, as they may have no financial resources at all. If their children brought them over to Canada in their later years, they may have no access to Canadian pensions, which makes them completely dependent on their children.

Health Impacts of Abuse

Age does make a difference with respect to identification and treatment of abuse. For example, some physical and psychological symptoms often associated with the aging process are similar in appearance to common consequences of abuse. This can result in misdiagnosis of older women's difficulties if the source of the problem is not identified. Symptoms such as depression, fatigue, anxiety, and confusion may be attributed to diminished capacity because of age rather than abuse (Wisconsin Coalition Against Domestic Violence, 1997, pp. 18-19; Hightower & Smith, 2002, pp. 55-56). Ongoing physical and psychological difficulties are found in stories from our respondents. As noted by one respondent, *"This extreme history of abuse has brought on several health challenges; ulcers, irritable bowel syndrome, stress, etc."*

Some women spoke of the responses of family physicians to their abusive situations. What often resulted was a prescription for medication. Some of the immigrant women have had less than supportive interventions from their family physicians. When an older Korean woman, abused by her husband and suffering from emotional stress, fear, and severe head aches, reported her problems to her family physician, he told her that she has no physical problem although he undertook no health assessment beyond listening to her complaints.

Impact on Adult Children of Witnessing Prior Abuse of Their Mothers

Some substantial recent work in the violence against women field has addressed the consequences for children of witnessing violence in the home (Sudermann & Jaffe, 1999; Edleson, 1999; Fantuzzo & Lindquist, 1989; Markowitz, 2001). The older women who told us of being abused while their children were young expressed great concern for the impact of this on their children. According to stories shared, children witnessed many of the situations of long-term abuse and situations of extreme violence. Particularly disturbing were the stories from women who have moved through several different abusive relationships with several children. The level and nature of the violence in these children's lives was serious. In some instances it is implied that the children were very afraid of their father or their mother's partner. It is clear they were aware of the violence. Some of the respondents told of instances when the children were also subjected to abuse. It is interesting that although they are clearly not familiar with the academic and clinical research on children who witness violence, these women express the same conclusions in similar terms. Many of these older women reported disturbing observations of their children's behaviour as adult partners and parents, thus extending the intergenerational impact to the third generation. This seems to lend support to the theory that violence and aggression are learned behaviours (DeKeseredy & MacLeod, 1997; Barnett et al., 1997).

Some of the women spoke sadly of being estranged from their adult children. One talked a great deal about her grown children, some of whom are in abusive relationships. Another woman talked of her son who turned to drugs at a young age and eventually moved back East. She is afraid that he will soon abuse his new wife; he recently told her that he finds himself treating his wife the way his dad treated her. On the other hand, there are instances in which the women speak of their children's resilience, and the fact that they managed to grow up to become strong and independent adults. Another woman shared her estrangement from her daughter saying,

I found out eventually that (my husband) had molested my five daughters from the time they were very young. My eldest daughter will have nothing to do with me because of her childhood. She says that I allowed her father to abuse her.

While some mothers said their adult children are not supportive of their leaving their abusive fathers in their later years, others mention adult children who had been supportive, indeed helped their mothers to leave, while staying in contact with their fathers. One woman, who had been a victim of long-term physical violence until she was removed from her situation by her daughter, spoke of the fact that this daughter and her other daughters were still in contact with their father. Another woman told of her children trying to persuade her to see their father again. It was suggested that adult children might fear they would become responsible for either their abused mother or abusive father. The fear of alienating their adult children's affection is one key factor that seemed to keep some older women in their abusive situations.

Impact of Leaving a Relationship in Later Life

The impacts of leaving a relationship in later life are associated with various problems and risks that are not present or are not the same for younger women. The potential losses include financial means and security, a home in which a woman may have invested a lifetime of care, and decades worth of the mementos and treasures that become increasingly precious in the later years of life.

Some older women need to find a place where they can take a dog or cat that has been their major source of support in recent years. An example of this involved a sixty-eight-year-old woman whose second husband took off and left her to deal with their bankruptcy. She had limited capability in English, and serious health problems. The only positive support in her life was a dog that she loved very much. Then service providers involved with her bankruptcy proceedings told her she should "get rid of the dog" to cut expenses.

In three of the stories the older women left their homes, and in two of these cases these were second relationships and the women owned the homes they left. In terms of social losses, it can mean leaving a neighborhood and familiar services and amenities that a woman may have used for many years. But it seems that the most overwhelming aspect of leaving that older women must cope with is accepting their losses when there does not seem any other option. To realize, after having tried to build a life, raise children, and care for a home that at the time when you should be enjoying some sense of accomplishment you have to leave to start over again from scratch, has a profound emotional impact. However, when she finds herself in later life in a relationship where her physical abuse is such that she is terrified of him, her options are very poor. As one woman said over the phone: *"I'm still very lonely. Can someone visit me?"*

The counsellors in these instances offered help in making local connections with community centres and with seniors' groups. The women were offered assistance in getting some counselling as well.

The women interviewed who had come to Canada in later life spoke of the isolation they experienced through being new in Canada, unable to speak English, and living in areas where no one else spoke their language. Those living with their sons' or daughters' families mentioned isolation and loneliness they experienced in their everyday family life.

Needs of Older Women Leaving Abusive Relationships

The needs of women who leave a relationship or a situation of abuse from a family member in later life are varied. Obviously they need either emergency or permanent housing, if they are faced with physically leaving their homes, and moving in with a child or other family members is not possible or suitable. Affordable rental housing for senior women, even those eligible for rent supplement (SAFER), is difficult if not virtually impossible to find in many places in British Columbia.

Leaving an abusive relationship is fraught with difficulties for a woman with disabilities. Health care or safety requirements may preclude many temporary and permanent housing options available to others, and she may have additional financial requirements. She may also need accommodation that enables her ease of access with her wheelchair. Most of the affordable housing supply and many shelters are in older structures that do not have the wider halls, doorways and other adaptations that are standard in newer structures. Three of the women who shared stories with us mentioned some physical disabilities, including one who has to use a motorized wheelchair. This woman was at the time of our meeting being harassed by a male neighbour in her apartment building.

As their first priority had to be safety, some of our respondents entered a women's shelter or moved in on a temporary basis with a family member. While some older women find women's shelters (transition houses) quite chaotic, some of our respondents said they had received great support and assistance from staff and fellow residents of these shelters. This may have been the first occasion in her life when she was able to share her experience with someone with the same problem. An elderly, perhaps isolated woman may need help with personal financial matters, such as applying for financial support and opening a bank account, as well as counselling and support services. Senior Citizen Counsellors in the province were particularly good at helping sort out financial matters, assisting in finding housing and other practical support services.

Counselling and group support is vital for many abused older women. While there are more of these support groups being developed in British Columbia, accessing this help in a small community or rural areas can be difficult for a variety of reasons. Maintaining confidentiality while accessing services in a smaller town is a major challenge. If there is counselling available in a small centre, often the woman seeking help knows the counsellor. This can be particularly difficult for an older woman. Much will depend on the relationships she and the counsellor have or have had in the past. Transportation can prove to be a major difficulty in urban and rural areas (Hemingway, 2001).

The reality for women in their fifties is they may need to find a job, but if they have never had a job, their chances of finding work are very poor. Women in such situations tell of being forced into minimum wage jobs. If these women have been isolated from employment by family responsibilities they face a terrible choice between two futures, abuse and economic security, or relative safety in poverty. In contrast, one of our respondents, a woman aged fifty-two who had recently left her relationship, said she had been able to plan her leaving over a long period of time.

> *Once our children left home, I upgraded my skills in night school and became more successful at my job so I was able to save for my escape and pay a lawyer to proceed.*

What we heard from all the women was that they wanted someone to listen to them, believe them, give practical advice and support, be trustworthy, and keep their confidence. Women identified practical advice and information from other women who had been in similar situations as being of major importance. Some women expressed concern and caution at the possibility of being referred to health services, as they feared this could result in being placed in an institution.

Who Helped, Who Didn't Help

In general, the women said little about sources of help, where they had sought it and who had responded. Three references were made to women's shelters or shelter staff, and one woman mentioned a helpful family physician. In two separate instances, older women's daughters took their mothers out of abusive situations. Each daughter went to her mother's house, packed her bags, and moved her mother into her, the daughter's, own home. Many of the women said that they had not shared with anyone the fact that they were being abused, so it makes some sense that there was little mention of help received.

Accessing help for those who have little or no English is an additional challenge. Cultural values may make it difficult to seek assistance. Older immigrant women often have no financial resources at all. If their children brought them over to Canada in their later years, they may have no access to Canadian pensions. The ten-year sponsorship rule is particularly problematic for older immigrant women.

Problems in getting help from government agencies were mentioned by some women but particularly by older immigrant women. This issue is reflected in the discussion with a group of counsellors working with immigrant older women. An older woman from Poland, who was interviewed with her counsellor translating, told how she came to Canada in a second marriage, sponsored by her husband. He became very abusive, and threatened to get her deported. She left him and stayed at a transition house. She got some assistance from legal aid and went to court to seek spousal support. The court process proved to be a nightmare for her. The Judge told her, "If you are that unhappy, go home to Poland." She has finally managed to get some support from income assistance.

Some women said that, in the past, when their abuse was known within the community, there was little response from neighbours or others. An older woman wrote that she had long suffered physical violence from both her husband and her brother-in-law, and had been hospitalized several times for her injuries. It would appear that her family doctor, and probably many others in the small community in which she lived, knew about this violence. Her life is very different now, thanks to the intervention of a relative.

Religious Beliefs

Three rather similar letters spoke at length of religious conviction and of being abused. They did not say that their abuse has ended; rather they imply or suggest that it has become unimportant. Since they found God, entered into a relationship with Him, nothing else matters. "He alone can heal the hurts and pain." It seems that their religious beliefs have given them comfort, and their faith in the next life makes unimportant whatever may be done to them in this life. Giesbrecht and Sevcik (2000) studied abused women (of all adult ages) in what they describe as "conservative evangelical subcultures." In this context, they concluded, the church functioned as an extended family system that could either minimize, deny, and enable abuse, or alternatively could provide much-needed social support, spiritual encouragement, and practical assistance. Some of the older women talked of turning to religion for support in the last couple of years. There is no evidence from their stories that it is the minister, or help from the congregation, that is the motivating factor behind this adoption of religion. It appears to be more connected to the ritual. There was no reference to any of the women asking the clergy for help. One woman said she was excommunicated from the Catholic Church because she left her abusive partner and then married a non-Catholic. Several immigrant women mentioned instances where their religious leaders were not helpful to them in dealing with their family problems.

Making Changes

It is never too late in life to make changes. Two of the women who shared their stories were over 80 years of age. Within the last five years they had made significant changes to their lives by leaving their abusive partners. Some of the respondents have indeed found happiness, in various degrees. For some, it is the first time in their life they have experienced independence and contentment. The women achieved this with assistance from friends, family, a shelter, a health provider, or a senior citizen counsellor. Some found safety and independence through their own strength and determination. These are women who demonstrated that "it is never too late to make a proper ending to earlier lives" (Pritchard, 2000, p. 112).

There are still many older women who we did not hear from who remain in abusive situations. Some respondents spoke of other older women they knew in similar situations. The stories received demonstrate how hard it is for an older woman to seek help to bring to an end an abusive relationship that may have continued for many years. This becomes particularly difficult if they serve as caregivers to their abusive partners, from whom they feel unable to leave because of a sense of loyalty, their marriage vows "to honour and obey until death do us part," family solidarity or loss of a home that they may have lived in for decades. For them happiness is still out of reach.

NEXT STEPS

We used what we had heard from abused older women to design a service delivery system that involved existing women's shelter resources, in particular trained staff with additional training in working with older women to serve as outreach workers, and volunteered safe homes for emergency refuge. This was a major recommendation in the project report, and funding followed for four pilot projects, three in British Columbia regions and one in the Yukon. A training curriculum on working with older women, an educational video and facilitator's study guide, and pamphlets for older women themselves and for those in occupations and professions that serve older women, were also funded (see www.bcysth.ca/projects/olderwomen.htm).

As we near the end of the three-year pilot project funding we can report that it has been successful in several respects. Funding has already been promised to continue the services in three of the areas, and possible expansion is being discussed. The broad outline of the service delivery model appears successful; though modifications will be recommended based on lessons learned from pilot testing and from suggestions by women served in the pilot sites, outreach workers and others in their communities. What we have heard from older abused women and their outreach workers supports and amplifies our earlier research results. The conceptual framework, gender plus age plus power and control, that guided our work is, we believe, supported by our results. Finally, and most importantly, a substantial number of older abused women have been supported in a process of assessing their safety and their options, making choices, and receiving practical and emotional support in getting on with their lives.

CONCLUSION

The intent of this participatory research process was to improve the response to abuse of older women by challenging existing beliefs and practices through personal contacts, the creation of new knowledge, and new materials that can lead to improvements in health policy development, implementation, and frontline practice.

All through their stories, women spoke of being emotionally abused, put down, denigrated and ridiculed. Older abused women need a safe environment, emotional support, an opportunity for sharing, education and information, a place to talk, interactions with other abused older women, the means for developing coping skills and decision-making abilities, and above all a way of shattering their isolation.

This research reinforces what is clear in the literature, that violence and abuse perpetrated by spouses and adult children have a negative impact on the health and well-being of older women. However, in recent years we have begun to recognize and address the intergenerational factors of violence. Older women shared stories of violence and abuse in their current and past lives and also in the lives of their parents and grandparents. The behavior of grandparents as well as parents has a significant effect on young children. When violence is present, it creates the facade that violence in families is the norm, perpetuating the cycle of violence.

Development of sound and effective strategies to end abuse within the family and promote safety needs to include input from victims and recognize the realities of their lives. Interdisciplinary approach based in qualitative research using victim insights and interdisciplinary cooperation between health and social service providers working with older adults and those who work primarily in the field of violence against women may result in better understanding and better outcomes for the women in question.

The life experience of many of the women who courageously shared their life experience of abuse demonstrates that for some women there is a continuum of violence across the life span, indeed from "Cradle to Grave."

REFERENCES

Aitken, L., & Griffin, G. (1996). *Gender Issues in Elder Abuse.* London: Sage.

American Association of Retired Persons (1994). *Survey of Services for Older Battered Women: Final Report.* Washington, DC: AARP.

Anike, L. (1999). *Report on Violence: Questionnaire on Violence and Abuse Against Older Women.* Older Women's Network, NSW, Australia.

Barnett, O. W., Miller-Perrin, C., & Perrin, R. D. (1997). *Family Violence Across the Lifespan: An Introduction.* Thousand Oaks: Sage.

Bowker, L. H. (1983). *Beating Wife Beating.* Toronto: Lexington.

Brandl, B., & Raymond, J. (1997). Unrecognized elder abuse victims. *Journal of Case Management, 6,* 62-68.

Browne, A. (1997). Violence in marriage: Until death do us part? In A. P. Cardarelli (Ed.), *Violence Between Intimate Partners.* Needham Heights, MA: Allyn & Bacon.

Cohen, L. (1984). *Small Expectations: Society's Betrayal of Older Women.* Toronto: McClelland and Stewart.

DeKeseredy, W. S., & MacLeod, L. (1997). *Woman Abuse: A Sociological Story.* Toronto: Harcourt Brace.

Edleson, J. (1999). Children's witnessing of adult domestic violence. *Journal of Interpersonal Violence, 14,* 8, 839-870.

Fantuzzo, J., & Lindquist, C. (1989). The effects of observing conjugal violence on children: A review and analysis of research methodology. *Journal of Family Violence, 4,* 77-94.

Giesbrecht, N., & Sevcik, I. (2000). The process of recovery and rebuilding among abused women in the conservative evangelical subculture. *Journal of Family Violence, 15* (3):229-248.

Harbison, J. (1999). The changing career of 'elder abuse and neglect' as a social problem in Canada: Learning from feminist frameworks? *Journal of Elder Abuse & Neglect, 11* (4), 59-80.

Heise, L.L., Pitanguy, J., & Germain, A. (1994). Violence against women: The hidden health burden. *World Bank Discussion Paper, 255,* Washington, DC: The Bank.

Hemingway, D. (2001). *Some Thoughts on the Needs, Difficulties, and Experiences of Abused Older Women Living in Northern, Rural or Remote Settings.* Unpublished.

Hightower, J., Smith, M.J., Ward-Hall, C. A., & Hightower, H. C. (1999). Meeting the needs of abused older women? A British Columbia and Yukon Transition House Survey. *Journal of Elder Abuse & Neglect, 11* (4), 39-58.

Hightower, J., Smith, M.J., & Hightower, H. C. (2001). *Silent and Invisible: A report on abuse and violence in the lives of older women in British Columbia and Yukon.* Vancouver: B.C./Yukon Society of Transition Houses.

Hightower, J., & Smith, M.J. (2002). *Silent and Invisible: What's Age Got to Do With It?* A handbook for Service Providers on Working with Abused Older Women in British Columbia and Yukon. Vancouver. B.C./Yukon Society of Transition Houses.

Jaffe, P.G., Russell, M., & Smith, M.J. (Eds.) (2000). *Creating a Legacy of Hope.* Vancouver: B.C./Yukon Society of Transition Houses.

Kappel, B., & Ramji, Z. (1998). *Study of Shelter Needs of Abused Older Women.* Toronto: Older Women's Network.

Markowitz, F. E. (2001). Attitudes and family violence: Linking intergenerational and cultural theories. *Journal of Family Violence, 16* (2), 205-218.

Mastrocola-Morris, E. (1989). *Woman Abuse: The Relationship Between Wife Assault and Elder Abuse.* Ottawa: National Clearinghouse on Family Violence.

Mears, J., & Sargent, M., (2002). *More than Survival: Project report two for professionals.* Sydney, Australia: University of Western Sydney.

Morgan Disney & Associates, Leigh Cupitt & Associates, & Council on the Ageing (2000). *Two Lives–Two Worlds: Older People and Domestic Violence* (2 Volumes). Canberra: Office of the Status of Women.

Mouton, C. P., & Espino, D. V. (1999). Health screening in older women. *American Family Physician,* April 1, 1999.

Mouton, C.P., Rodabough, R.J. et al. (2004). Prevalence and three-year incidence of abuse among postmenopausal women. In *American Journal of Public Health, 94* (4): 605-12.

National Centre on Elder Abuse (2000). Violence against women act adds older women provisions. Washington: NCEA: *Newsletter,* Nov 2000, 3-4.

Nudelman, J. (1999). Building Bridges between Domestic Violence Advocates and Health Care Providers. National Resource Center on Domestic Violence. http://www.vawnet.org/vnl/library/general/bcs6_hc.htm

Older Women's Long-term Survival Society (n.d.). *Older Women Survivors: A Video and Handbook for and About Older Women who have Survived Abuse.* Alberta.

Pritchard, J. (2000). *The Needs of Older Women: Services for Victims of Elder Abuse and Other Abuse.* Bristol, UK: The Policy Press.

Sacco, V.F. (1990). Elder abuse policy: An assessment of categoric approaches. In Roesch, R., Dutton, D.G., & Sacco, V.F. (Eds.), *Family Violence: Perspectives on Treatment, Research, and Policy.* Burnaby, BC: B.C. Institute on Family Violence.

Sargent, M., & Mears, J. (2000). *Older Women Speak Up.* Campbelltown, NSW: University of Western Sydney.

Sargent, M., & Mears, J. (2002). *More than Survival: Project report one for older women*. Sydney, Australia: University of Western Sydney.

Schaffer, J. (1999). Older and isolated women and domestic violence project. *Journal of Elder Abuse & Neglect, 11* (1), 59-73.

School of Public Health, Johns Hopkins University (1999). Ending violence against women. *Population Reports, Series L*, Number 11, December 1999.

Scott, M., McKie, L., Morton, S., Seddon S., Wasoff, S., & Fran, S. (2004). *Older Women and Domestic Violence in Scotland*. Health Scotland, Woodburn House Edinburgh.

Seaver, C. (1996). Muted lives: Older battered women. *Journal of Elder Abuse & Neglect, 8*, 3-21.

Sedger, R. (2001). Is it aged abuse or domestic violence? Australian domestic & family violence clearinghouse. *Newsletter, 9*, 3-4.

Speltz, K., & Raymond, J. (2000). Elder abuse, including domestic violence in later life. *Wisconsin Lawyer, 73* (9).

Statistics Canada (1998). *Family Violence in Canada: A Statistical Profile*. Ottawa: Statistics Canada.

Stewart, D. (2000). *Older Women and the Violence Against Women in Relationship Policy in British Columbia*. New Westminster, BC: B.C. Coalition to Eliminate Abuse of Seniors.

Sudermann, M., & Jaffe, P. (1999). *A Handbook for Health and Social Service Providers and Educators on Children Exposed to Woman Abuse/Family Violence*. Ottawa: Health Canada, Family Violence Prevention Unit.

United Nations (1993). *Declaration on the Elimination of Violence against Women*. General Assembly, 85th plenary meeting 20 December 1993 48/104.

Vinton, L. (1992). Battered women's shelters and older women: The Florida experience. *Journal of Family Violence, 7*, 63-72.

Vinton, L. (1997). *Questions and Answers about Older Battered Women*. Florida Department of Elder Affairs. http://www.state.fl.us/does/battwomen.html

Vinton, L. (1998). A nationwide survey of domestic violence shelters' programming for older women. *Violence Against Women, 4*, 559-571.

WHO/INPEA (2002). *Missing Voices: Views of Older Persons on Elder Abuse*. Geneva: World Health Organization.

Wisconsin Coalition Against Domestic Violence (1997). *Developing Services for Older Abused Women: A Guide for Domestic Abuse Programs*. Madison, WI: Wisconsin Coalition Against Domestic Violence.

Effects of Dependency
on Compliance Rates
Among Elder Abuse Victims
at the New York City Department
for the Aging, Elderly Crime Victim's Unit

Mebane E. Powell, MSW
Jacquelin Berman, PhD

SUMMARY. A study was conducted at the New York City Department for the Aging Elderly Crime Victim's Unit (ECVU) to examine the relationship between dependency and compliance rates. Dependency was defined by the total score for each case on the Victim Dependency Scale and Abuser Dependency Scale. Compliance was defined as the act of accepting a referral and compliance rates were determined by counting the total number of referrals the victim accepted. Findings indicated that the only factor associated with compliance rates was if the abuser had a mental illness/substance abuse problem. If the abuser did have this problem, the victim was significantly more likely to accept a referral for services as compared to victims whose abusers did not have a mental illness/substance abuse problem ($t = -2.774$, $df = 36.899$, $p < .01$). The

[Haworth co-indexing entry note]: "Effects of Dependency on Compliance Rates Among Elder Abuse Victims at the New York City Department for the Aging, Elderly Crime Victim's Unit." Powell, Mebane E., and Jacquelin Berman. Co-published simultaneously in *Journal of Gerontological Social Work* (The Haworth Press, Inc.) Vol. 46, No. 3/4, 2006, pp. 229-247 ; and: *Elder Abuse and Mistreatment: Policy, Practice, and Research* (ed: M. Joanna Mellor, and Patricia Brownell) The Haworth Press, Inc., 2006, pp. 229-247. Single or multiple copies of this article are available for a fee from The Haworth Document Delivery Service [1-800-HAWORTH, 9:00 a.m. - 5:00 p.m. (EST). E-mail address: docdelivery@haworthpress.com].

authors offer explanations as to why this research was important and the implications it has on future research. *[Article copies available for a fee from The Haworth Document Delivery Service: 1-800-HAWORTH. E-mail address: <docdelivery@haworthpress.com> Website: <http://www.HaworthPress. com> © 2006 by The Haworth Press, Inc. All rights reserved.]*

KEYWORDS. Elder abuse, dependency, compliance, mental illness, substance abuse

Elder abuse is defined as "an all-inclusive term representing all types of mistreatment or abusive behavior toward older adults" (Wolf, 2000, p. 7). Elder abuse has been identified as a growing problem not only due to the increasing number of people who are coming into the 60 and older age group but also because for the first time in the year 2025, the number of people age 60 and older will match that of people age 0-14 globally (United Nations Population Division: World Population Aging: 1950-2050).

The New York City Department for the Aging, the largest Area Agency on Aging in the United States, houses an Elderly Crime Victim's Unit (ECVU). Suspected and/or confirmed physical, emotional, financial, and sexual abuse, as well as acts of neglect can be reported to the ECVU by anyone in the community. The ECVU acts as an information and referral source for all cases of elder abuse, including those with and without capacity.

According to the New York City Department for the Aging, New York City in 2000 was home to 39.1% of all people over the age of 60 in New York State (New York City Department for the Aging: Quick Facts, 2003). In New York State "estimates on incidence and prevalence of elder abuse and neglect have ranges from 3 to 40 per thousand depending on the definition used and the population studied" (Brownell, Welty & Brennan, 2001-2003, ¶ 1). Due to the lack of elder abuse studies in New York City, the prevalence and incidence rates of elder abuse in New York City are impossible to determine. What is known is that between January 1, 1999 and July 31, 2002, the Department for the Aging opened 2,472 elder abuse cases (Mayor's Office to Combat Domestic Violence, 2002). It can be expected that as the number of elderly age sixty and older in New York City continues to grow, so will the incidence and prevalence of elder abuse (Wolf, 2000). Thus, there is a pressing need for research in the area of elder abuse, especially in New York City.

RATIONALE OF STUDY

To date the literature has shown that the victim reported in studies is typically living with the abuser and has some sort of mental or cognitive deficiency (National Research Council, 2003). The jury is still out on if variables such as race, gender, age, and physical impairment of the older victim are significantly associated with elder abuse (National Research Council, 2003). As noted by the National Research Counsel "no survey of the U.S. population has ever been undertaken to provide a national estimate for the occurrence of any form of elder mistreatment; the magnitude of the problem–among community-dwelling elders, as well as those residing in long-term care facilities–is basically unknown" (National Research Council, 2003, p. xiii) therefore, the profile of the typical victim and abuser is still largely unknown.

Previous studies (Wolf et al., 1982) noted that abusers tended to be financially dependent on the victim (as cited in National Research Council, 2003). Other studies (Pillemer, 1986; Wolf & Pillemer, 1989) have found that abusers were also financially dependent on victims and dependent on victims for housing as well (as cited in National Research Council, 2003). On the other hand, the following studies (Bristowe & Collins, 1989; Homer & Gilleard, 1990; Phillips, 1983; Pillemer, 1985; Wolf & Pillemer, 1989; Pillemer & Finkelhor, 1989; Pillemer & Suitor, 1992; Reis & Nahmiash, 1997) examined the dependency of victims on the abuser and did not find greater dependency on abusers by victims when compared with nonvictims (as cited in National Research Council, 2003).

Due to the fact that the body of literature on elder abuse recognizes the dependency of the abuser on the victim as a substantiated risk factor for elder abuse, the authors wanted to explore how the issue of dependency of the abuser on the victim as well as the victim on the abuser may impact the victim's acceptance rate of referrals (compliance).

RESEARCH QUESTION AND HYPOTHESES

This research study seeks to answer the question "At the New York City Department for the Aging, Elderly Crime Victim's Unit, does the compliance rate in elders who are reported as being victims of abuse differ depending on the level of dependency of the abuser on the victim and/or the level of dependency of the victim on the abuser?" To measure the level of dependency of the abuser on the victim and the victim on the abuser, the authors created a Dependency Scale based on a previous study conducted in New York City that asked victims about their dependency on the abuser (see Appendix A & B).

The term compliance "refers to the tendency of the individual to go along with propositions, requests or instructions, for some immediate instrumental gain" (Gudjonsson, 1992, p. 137) (as cited in Gudjonsson & Sigurdsson, 2003, p. 117). There are some studies that measure compliance in terms of a behavioral response to a given situation (Gudjonsson & Sigurdsson, 2003; Gudjonsson, Sigurdsson, Brynjolfsdottir, & Hreinsdottir, 2002). In each of these studies, the Gudjonsson Compliance Scale (GCS) (Gudjonsson & Sigurdsson, 2003) that measures "the tendency to conform to requests made by others, particularly people in authority, in order to please them or to avoid conflict and confrontation" (p. 118) is what has been used to measure a person's compliance.

While several studies did examine compliance in a social work realm, the researchers studied subjects in mental health hospitals and settings and operationally defined compliance as the subject's willingness to following through with the doctor's referral to mental health clinics (Griffith, 2001; Jennings & Ball, 1982; Krulee & Hales, 1988). In the study conducted by Griffith (2001) compliance was not viewed in any theoretical framework, nor were outside social factors examined in terms of affecting referral compliance. In a study by Jennings and Ball (1982) that examined a patient's willingness to use the Civilian Health and Medical Program of Uniformed Services, findings indicated that socioeconomic status did not significantly impact rates of compliance. Krulee and Hales (1988) examined the referral patterns of patients in a general hospital psychiatry outpatient clinic and found factors associated with higher compliance rates included being married, having the referral process initiated by the therapist, and for a small group of patients, receiving a list of potential psychotherapists. With the lack in research centered on social work in community based organizations and compliance, one cannot assume that what applies in the medical setting applies in the community. Thus, there is a great need for researching compliance in community based social work settings.

This author notes that there is also a body of literature that denotes a set of risk factors as contested risk factors (National Research Council, 2003). Thus, for the purpose of this study only those risk factors that have been "validated by substantial evidence, for which there is unanimous or near unanimous support from a number of studies" (National Research Council, 2003, p. 92) and for which data can be gathered from the ECVU intake form will be considered as covariates to dependency and compliance rates. These factors include dementia of the victim, alcohol use, and mental illness.

In order to determine what effect the presence of aforementioned risk factors had in impacting compliance rate and dependency levels, the risk factors of mental health/substance abuse issues were taken into account for the victim and the abuser. Based on the literature review the following hypotheses were developed:

1. There is a significant difference in compliance rates based on the victim's Victim Dependency Scale Score.
2. There is a significant difference in compliance rates based on the victim's Abuser Dependency Scale Score.
3. There is a significant difference in compliance rates based on the abuser's mental illness/substance abuse status.
4. There is a significant difference in compliance rates based on the victim's mental health status.

METHOD

Study Design

In order to answer the research question, and test the hypotheses the author conducted a study at the New York City Department for the Aging's Elderly Crime Victim's unit (ECVU). The study utilized a cross-sectional design that took a snapshot of the ECVU's elder abuse victims at a single point in time, January to March, 2004. Information about the ECVU's elder abuse victims was gathered from the intake form. Information about dependency was gathered from the case managers' point-of-view when the case manager completed the Dependency Scale (see Appendix A) for each elder abuse case that was closed between January and March 2004. The research was associational, in that "statistically significant correlation coefficients between and among relevant phenomena," dependency and compliance, "[were] sought and interpreted" (Mauch & Birch, 1983, p. 70).

Study Population

A total sample of 95 elder abuse cases were closed between January and March 2004 at the New York City Department for the Aging, Elderly Crime Victim's Unit and all 95 closed cases were included in this study. The 95 cases were assessed by their assigned case manager who filled out the Dependency Scale for each closed case based on all information gathered about the closed case. The data from the closed cases was entered into a "client/abuser" database with all identifiers having been removed and was then sent to the authors for analysis.

VARIABLES

Descriptives

The variables of age (exact age), sex (male/female), and race/ethnicity (White, Black, Hispanic, Asian, Other) were taken from the intake form for both the victim and the abuser. Each variable was represented in the data file with appropriate codes and labels.

Dependent Variable

The dependent variable of compliance was defined as the act of verbally accepting a referral from a New York City Department for the Aging, Elderly Crime Victims Unit's case manager to either an in-house or an outside community based organization. This act of verbal acceptance is noted as a nominal variable on the intake form under the question "Is client willing to accept any of the following services: Order of Protection, Eviction, Lock Replacement, Long Term Counseling, DVO/Police Intervention, District Attorney's Office, Health Care, Mobile Crisis/Mental Health, Financial Assistance, Case Management, Housing, Mental Hygiene Warrant, Other?" A count of the total number of referrals (0-12) accepted by the elder abuse victim from the ECVU was conducted for each victim and indicated in the data file by the variable "Yesref."

Independent Variable

Construction of Scale. Prior to the development of the Dependency Scale, approval was granted from the appropriate sources to use and modify the original dependency scale (Davis, Median, & Avitabile, 2001) used in the following study conducted by the National Institute of Justice (see Appendix B).

The authors' Dependency Scale (see Appendix A) consisted of two Likert scales. The first scale, Abuser Dependency Scale (ADS), examined how dependent the abuser is on the victim and used a Likert scale with values ranging from 1 to 5, with 1 being "not at all dependent" and 5 being "completely dependent." The second scale, Victim Dependency Scale (VDS), examined how dependent the victim is on the abuser using a Likert scale with values ranging from 1 to 5 with 1 being "not at all dependent" and 5 being "completely dependent."

Instructions. Instructions for the scale were administered verbally by the authors during the case manager meeting on January 16, 2004. Each case manager in the ECVU was told by the authors to complete the Dependency Scale using all information from the closed case that they had gathered. For both the ADS and the VDS if the case manager in the ECVU did not know what to rate a person on a particular question, there was the option of choosing "don't know" for the question. However, case managers at the ECVU were encourage not to use this option unless absolutely necessary.

Scoring. For both scales in the Dependency Scale, the higher the scale score, the higher the level of the dependency of the victim on the abuser and/or the abuser on the victim, from the case manager's point-of-view. The level of dependency for the victim was defined by adding all the scores of VDS questions 1-6 in SPSS. Questions that were coded as "don't know" were not included in the total scale score. The VDS maximum scale score was 30. The level of dependency for the abuser is defined by adding all the scores of ADS questions 1-4 in SPSS. Questions that were coded as "don't know" were not included in the total scale score. The maximum scale score for the ADS scale was 20.

COVARIATES

Mental Illness/Substance Abuse Problem

A series of dichotomous variables were constructed whenever there was indication on the intake form that the victim had "Indicated problem area" or "professionally diagnosed" for any of the following variables: alcohol abuse, drug abuse, MICA, confusion/disorientation, forgetfulness, dementia, mental illness. These new variables were recoded under the variable "victimmentalyesno" as "yes"/"1" to indicate the presence of mental illness/substance abuse issues. Mental illness of the abuser was defined the same way as it was for the victim and recoded under the variable "abusermentalyesno."

DESCRIPTION OF SAMPLE

Profile of the Victim

There were a total of 95 closed cases. The data collected for the purpose of this study indicate that of the victims of elder abuse that were reported to DFTA's ECVU 36.5% (n = 34) are between the ages of 80-89, 31% (n = 29) between 70-79, 19.4% (n = 18) between 60-69, 11.8% (n = 11) between 90-99, 1.1% (n = 1) 100 years or older, with 2 people missing information. In terms of gender, the majority are female (84.0%, n = 79) with only one person missing information. For the variable race/ethnicity, 50.0% (n = 36) of the victims are

Black, 31.9% (n = 23) are White, 9.7% (n = 7) are Hispanic, 8.4% (n = 6) are coded as Other, and 23 people have missing information. The majority 83.7% (n = 77) live with another adult who is typically an adult child (40.7%, n = 35) and over one-third of the cases reported to the ECVU are reported by family members (37.6%, n = 35). Case managers that were able to gather information on the mental/physical health of the victim found that the majority 87.5% (n = 70) did not have alcohol or drug problems, 38.5% (n = 30) reported confusion as an indicated problem area or professionally diagnosed problem area, 42.3% (n = 33) reported forgetfulness, and 29.9% (n = 23) of the victims reported dementia as an indicated problem area or professionally diagnosed problem area.

Profile of the Abuser

The data collected for the purpose of this study indicate that of the abusers that were reported to DFTA's ECVU 26.2% (n = 16) are between the ages of 40-49, 19.7% (n = 12) are between the ages of 30-39, 18.0% (n = 11) between 50-59, 11.5% (n = 7) between 20-29, 9.8% (n = 6) between 15-19, 6.6% (n = 4) between 60-69, 4.9% (n = 3) between 70-79, 3.3% (n = 2) between 80-89 and 34 were missing information. In terms of relationship to the victim, 39.5% (n = 34) are children of the victim, 22.1% (n = 19) are non-relatives of the victim (e.g., girlfriend of the victim's son, home attendant), 14.0% (n = 12) are a relative other than a grandchild, child, sibling or spouse, 11.6% (n = 10) are a spouse/domestic partner, 10.5% (n = 9) are an adult grandchild, 2.3% (n = 2) are siblings and 9 are missing information. Regarding race/ethnicity, the majority 60.4% (n = 29) are Black, 27.1% (n = 13) are White, 4.2% (n = 2) are Hispanic and 8.3% (n = 4) are coded as Other, and 47 are missing information. The gender of the abusers is equally split between women (50.0%, n = 40) and men (50.0%, n = 40) with 15 people missing information. Case managers that were able to gather information on the mental/physical health of the abuser found that 26.6% (n = 17) have alcohol problems, 22.7% (n = 15) have drug problems, and 4.7% (n = 3) are reported as MICA clients. Approximately one-fourth of the abusers were reported as having a mental illness as a professionally diagnosed/indicated problem area (24.3%, n = 15). Information gathered about the abuser from various sources indicated that the majority of abusers 84.4% (n = 54) were not reported as having confusion as an indicated problem area or professionally diagnosed problem area, 84.4% (n = 54) did not report forgetfulness, and 83.9% (n = 52) of abusers were not reported as having dementia as an indicated problem area or professionally diagnosed problem area.

FINDINGS

Hypothesis 1

A bivariate correlation was conducted between compliance rates and the Victim Dependency Scale Score (see Table 1). A negative relationship between compliance rates and the victim dependency scale was found; however, the correlation was not significant between the two variables, resulting in a failure to reject the null hypothesis.

Hypothesis 2

A bivariate correlation was conducted between compliance rates and the Victim's Abuser Dependency Scale Score (see Table 1). Results showed that while a positive relationship between compliance rates and Abuser Dependency Scale Scores existed, the correlation was not significant between the two variables, resulting in a failure to reject the null hypothesis.

Hypothesis 3

Due to the independent variable (abuser's mental illness/substance abuse status) being dichotomous, a t-test was conducted between compliance rates and the abuser's mental illness/substance abuser status (see Table 2). Results indicated that there is a significant difference between the mean number of referrals accepted (compliance rate) between the victims whose abusers have mental illness/substance abuse issues versus victims whose abusers do not have mental illness/substance abuse issues, thus resulting in a failure to accept the null hypothesis ($t = -2.774$, $df = 36.899$, $p < .01$).

TABLE 1. Results of Bivariate Correlations for Hypothesis 1: There is a significant difference in compliance rates based on victim's Victim Dependency Scale Score and Hypothesis 2: There is a significant difference in compliance rates based on the victim's Abuser Dependency Scale Score.

	Pearson's r	p-value	N
Hypothesis 1	−.019	.865	86
Hypothesis 2	.141	.193	87

TABLE 2. Results of T-test for Hypothesis 3: There is a significant difference in compliance rates based on the abuser's mental illness/substance abuse status and Hypothesis 4: There is a significant difference in compliance rates based on the victim's mental health status.

	t-value	df	p-value
Hypothesis 3	−2.774	36.899	.009
Hypothesis 4	−.615	93	.540

Hypothesis 4

Due to the independent variable (victim's mental health status) being dichotomous, a t-test was conducted between compliance rates and the victim's mental health status (see Table 2). Results indicated that there is no significant difference between the mean number of referrals accepted (compliance rate) between those victims who have mental health issues and those victims who do not have mental health issues, thus resulting in a failure to reject the null hypothesis.

DISCUSSION

The purpose of this study was to gather information on the levels of dependency of the elder abuse victim on the abuser and the abuser on the elder abuse victim to better understand whether dependency affects the elder abuse victim's acceptance of referrals when taking the influence of the background of the abuser and victim into account. Based on this study's hypotheses and subsequent findings, only hypothesis 3–there is a difference in compliance rates based on the abuser's mental illness/substance abuse status–was supported ($t = -2.774$, $df = 36.899$, $p < .01$). Thus, indicating that elder abuse victims whose abusers have a mental illness/substance abuse problem are significantly more likely to accept referrals than those elder abuse victims whose abusers do not have a mental illness/substance abuse problem.

Based on these findings, a second stage of analysis was performed to provide more information about the independent variable mental illness/substance abuse of the abuser. This author examined the question "Of the closed cases assessed for dependency by case managers at the New York City Department for the Aging, are there differences between the groups of abusers who have a mental illness/substance abuse issue and those that do not on such variables as age, race, gender, type of abuse reported, and dependency levels?"

When exploring the two groups, victims whose abusers have substance abuse/mental illness and victims whose abusers do not, there were no significant differences in the victim's age (t = .934, df = 91, p = .353), race (χ^2 = 1.783, p = .619) and gender (χ^2 = .025, p = .875). Similarly, there were no significant differences between the two groups of abusers on the variables of age (t = .006, df = 59, p = .995), race (χ^2 = 1.061, p = .786) and gender (χ^2 = 5.296, p = .071). When exploring the type of abuse reported by the two groups of victims there were no significant differences in the amount of financial, physical, and sexual abuse reported. However, there were differences in the amount of psychological/emotional abuse and acts of neglect.

Approximately 96.9% of victims whose abusers have a substance abuse/mental illness issue report that the abuser is psychologically/emotionally abusive compared to 68% of victims whose abusers do not have substance abuse/mental illness issues (χ^2 = 9.900, p < .01). On the other hand, 15.6% of victims whose abusers do have substance abuse/mental illness issues reported that the abuser is actively/passively neglecting them compared to 46% of victims whose abusers do not have substance abuse/mental illness issues (χ^2 = 8.006, p < .01).

When investigating differences between the two groups of abusers and the ratings by case managers on the dependency scale it was found that abusers who have substance abuse/mental illness issues are significantly more dependent on the victim than abusers who do not have substance abuse/mental illness issues (t = −4.293, df = 85, p < .001). Similarly, victims of abuse who have substance abuse/mental illness issues are significantly less likely to be dependent on the abuser than victims whose abusers do not have substance abuse/mental illness issues (t = 2.680, df = 80.513, p < .009).

When the ADS scale was examined by each individual question for any significant differences between the two groups of abusers, it was found that abusers who have a substance abuse/mental illness issue are significantly more likely to be dependent on the victim for a place to live, expenses, cooking and cleaning (t = −5.031, df = 81.725, p < .001; t = −3.631, df = 70, p <.01; t = −4.225, df = 78, p < .001, respectively) from the case manager's point-of-view.

When the VDS scale was examined by each individual question for any significant differences between the two groups of abusers, it was found that victims of abusers who do not have substance abuse/mental illness issues are more dependent on the abuser for food/clothing/transportation costs, meal preparation, cleaning, and taking medications/walks/dress/bathe (t = 2.380, df = 75.061, p < .05; t = 3.892, df = 79.641, p < .001; t = 3.726, df = 78.999, p < .001; t = 3.477, df = 81.886, p < .01, respectively) from the case manager's point-of-view.

Dependency Scale

The construction of the dependency scale was discussed previously in the Methods section. In order to assess the reliability of the VDS and ADS scales, SPSS was used to calculate Cronbach's Alpha along with inter-item correlations for the VDS and ADS (see Table 3). The high inter-item correlations in the VDS between cleaning and medications as well as meals and medications, and cleaning and meals; and in the ADS between cooking and expenses suggests that these items could be combined in future studies where the sole purpose of the scale is for case managers to rate the dependency of the victim on the abuser. However, if this scale is used to ascertain dependency of the victim on the abuser and the abuser on the victim with the sole purpose of guiding case managers to offer certain services, then these items should not be combined for future studies examining the scale in the context of being a guide to services offered.

LIMITATIONS

The primary limitation of this study is that due to the amount of missing data for some of the demographics, such as race of the abuser and exact age of

TABLE 3. Cronbach's Alpha and Inter-Item Correlations for the Abuser Dependency Scale and the Victim Dependency Scale.

Abuser Dependency Scale			
Cronbach's Alpha = .833			
	Question 1	Question 2	Question 3
Question 2	.922	------	------
Question 3	.190	.187	------
Question 4	.841	.767	.143

Victim Dependency Scale					
Cronbach's Alpha = .932					
	Question 1	Question 2	Question 3	Question 4	Question 5
Question 2	.769	-------	------	------	------
Question 3	.494	.761	------	------	------
Question 4	.489	.753	.979	------	------
Question 5	.731	.758	.537	.525	------
Question 6	.478	.718	.951	.973	.511

the abuser, assumptions that this data are representative of DFTA clients and can provide a basis for client and/or abuser profiles cannot be made with any degree of certainty.

The second limitation of the study is the relatively small sample size of 95 closed cases. Ideally, a replication of this study with a larger sample size over a longer timeframe would be needed before any generalizations or conclusions from this study could be made about DFTA ECVU victims and abusers and compliance rates.

The third limitation of this study is the inability to measure levels of dependency directly from the elder abuse victim. As noted by Widlack, Greenley, and McKee (1992) "case managers can never know the client's condition directly; they can ascertain it only by inference from observation, by report of the client or by hearsay" (p. 507). Thus, the case managers in this study lack the ability to verify any of the victims' levels of dependency on the abuser and vice-versa. However, using case manager reports to conduct research on various aspects of the client is becoming an increasingly common method (Widlack, Greenley, & McKee, 1992). There are several benefits to using case manager reports and Widlack, Greenley, and McKee (1992) list the following: (1) Case managers have broad information on the client; (2) Case managers' gathering of information is less costly than a researcher gathering the same information; (3) Case managers make good respondents; (4) Case managers are less likely to drop out of the study and cause loss of cases; (5) Case managers, in some instances, are thought to be better sources of information when clients may be reluctant to answer sensitive questions.

IMPLICATIONS FOR PRACTICE AND RECOMMENDATIONS FOR FUTURE RESEARCH

The dependency of the victim on the abuser and the abuser on the victim as rated by the case manager was found to be unrelated to the amount of services the victim accepts. Only one aspect of the abuser, mental illness/substance abuse issues, had a significant relationship to the number of services a victim accepts. Since there is little research to date to state if this finding is consistent with other research findings that examine dependency and compliance rate of elder abuse victims, statements about these findings must be taken within the context of this study.

Findings of this study can be important in developing future models of the Dependency Scale to be used to examine compliance rates or as a guide to offering services. As demonstrated in this study, the factor that was associated with compliance rate was not dependency levels but whether the abuser had a mental illness/substance abuse issue. Analyzing the dependency scale for victims whose abusers have these issues and for those abusers who do not have these issues may be beneficial in determining if there are differences between these two groups in terms of dependency and compliance rates.

The finding that the presence of mental illness/substance abuse problems of the abuser is significantly associated with the victim being more likely to accept a referral requires further investigation before making any assumptions as to why this was found. One could speculate that this may have been found because those victims whose abusers have these issues were offered more services than those victims whose abusers do not have these issues. However, more research is needed in this area before determining the impact of this finding and should be a natural next step in following up this research study. If it is found that victims of abusers who have mental illness/substance abuse issues are more likely to be offered more services than those victims whose abusers do not have this issue, this finding could significantly impact the way services are offered at DFTA's ECVU and how case managers are trained in terms of how to offer services.

Similarly, the first finding that those victims whose abusers have substance abuse/mental illness issues do not differ on age, race, and gender is interesting in that it fails to support the often noted theory that abusers go after older, more frail and female individuals and that abusers are often male. The second finding that victims of abusers with substance abuse/mental illness issues report more instances of psychological/emotional abuse coincides with the finding that case managers report these same victims as being significantly less dependent on the abuser and the abuser being significantly more dependent on the victim. The third finding that victims of abusers who do not have a substance abuse/mental illness issue report more instances of active/passive neglect coincides with the finding that case managers report these same victims as being significantly more dependent on the abuser and the abuser significantly less dependent on the victim.

The aforementioned findings indicate that from the case manager's view-points there are clearly two distinct groups of abusers. The two groups of abusers, those with substance abuse/mental illness issues and those without these issues, lend themselves to further discussion. It has been well documented that abusers with substance abuse issues oftentimes psychologically and emotionally manipulate the people around them in order to gain the money or necessary resources to support their abuse/addiction. Similarly, those with mental illness issues may or may not use drugs and often, due to their mental illness either not being treated properly or not having been diagnosed, may lack the ability to be able to distinguish between appropriate and inappropriate behaviors. On the other hand, it has often been noted in elder abuse literature that abusers tend to be children of the elderly who see their parents as vulnerable due to being older, frailer and less able to take care of themselves. While this study does indicate that the elderly victim is more dependent on the abuser, from the case manager's point of view, this study did not find that these victims tend to be older than those victims of abusers who do have a substance abuse/mental illness issue. Furthermore, there is a need to examine more closely the victims of abuse whose abusers have a substance abuse/mental illness issue, since the authors in this limited study found that these victims were significantly more likely to want help than those whose abusers do not have this issue.

For future studies the authors believe that it is essential to start investigating the term "abusers" not as an all-encompassing category, but as at least four different groups: (1) Abusers who do not have any reported or current substance abuse issues; (2) Abusers who do not have any reported or current mental illness issues; (3) Abusers who do not have both 1 and 2; and (4) Abusers who have both 1 and 2. The authors believe that in doing so, it will be easier to start formulating typologies of abusers and this will lead to being able to determine if an elder is at risk for experiencing elder abuse. The need to start distinguishing groups of abusers and typologies of abusers is not new. As noted by Ramsey-Klawsnik (2000) five types of offenders were postulated based on her experiences in conducting forensic investigation; they were: (1) the overwhelmed; (2) the impaired; (3) the narcissistic; (4) the domineering and (5) the sadistic. These typologies were formulated to illustrate the complexities of those that abuse the elderly. Similarly, this author's limited study found that when using the term "abuser" to illustrate all possible types of abusers that valuable findings may be lost and embedded in results that may or may not support a stated hypothesis.

REFERENCES

Bristowe, E. & Collins, J.B. (1989). Family-mediated abuse of non-institutionalized elder men and women living in British Columbia. *Journal of Elder Abuse & Neglect 1*(1):45-54.

Brownell, P., Welty, A., & Brennan, M. (2001-2003). Elder Abuse and Neglect. In *Project 2015*, New York State Office for the Aging, Retrieved November 9, 2003 from http://www.aging.state.ny.us/explore/project2015/articles.htm.

Davis, R. C., Median, J., & Avitabile, N. (2001). *National Institute of Justice: Effectiveness of a Joint Police Response to Elder Abuse in Manhattan [New York City], New York, 1996-1997.* (Publication No. 3130). Retrieved September 20, 2003 from ICPSR website http://www.icpsr.umich.edu/.

Griffith, K. (2001). Compliance with mental health referrals: Does it increase over time? University of North Carolina at Charlotte: *Undergraduate Journal of Psychology, 14*, 1-4. Retrieved September 25, 2003 from http://www.psych.uncc.edu/ UJOP2001.pdf.

Gudjonsson, G., & Sigurdsson, J. F. (2003). The relationship of compliance with coping strategies and self-esteem. *European Journal of Psychological Assessment, 19*(2), 117-123.

Gudjonsson, G., Sigurdsson, J. F., Brynjolfsdottir, B., & Hreinsdottir, H. (2002). The relationship of compliance with anxiety, self-esteem, paranoid thinking, and anger. *Psychology, Crime & Law, 8*, 145-153.

Homer, A.C., & Gilleard, C. (1990). Abuse of elderly people by their caregivers. *British Medical Journal 31*(6765):1359-1362.

Jennings, R., & Ball, J. (1982). Patient compliance with CHAMPUS mental health referrals. *Professional Psychology: Research & Practice, 13*(20), 172-173.

Krulee, D., & Hales, R. (1988). Compliance with psychiatric referrals from a general hospital psychiatry outpatient clinic. *General Hospital Psychiatry, 10*(5), 339-345.

Mauch, J. E., & Birch, J. W. (1983). *Guide to the Successful Thesis and Dissertation.* New York: Marcel Dekker, Inc.

Mayor's Office to Combat Domestic Violence (2002). *New York City Domestic Violence Fact Sheet*, December, 2002.

National Research Council. (2003). *Elder Mistreatment: Abuse, Neglect, and Exploitation in an Aging America.* Panel to Review Risk and Prevalence of Elder Abuse and Neglect. Richard J. Bonnie and Robert B. Wallace (Eds.). Committee on National Statistics and Committee on Law and Justice, Division of Behavioral and Social Sciences and Education. Washington, DC: The National Academies Press.

New York City Department for the Aging: *Quick Facts*, July, 2003.

Phillips, L.R. (1983). Abuse and neglect of the frail elderly at home: An exploration of theoretical relationships. *Journal of Advanced Nursing* 8:379-392.

Pillemer, K.A. (1985). The dangers of dependency: New findings on domestic violence against the elderly. *Social Problems 33*(2):146-158.

Pillemer, K. A. (1986) Risk factors in elder abuse: Results from a case-control study. In *Elder Abuse: Conflict in the Family*, K.A. Pillemer and R.S. Wolf, eds. Dover, DE: Auburn House Publishing Company.

Pillemer, K.A., & Finkelhor, D. (1989). Causes of elder abuse: Caregiver stress versus problem relatives. *American Journal of Orthopsychiatry 59*: 179-187.

Pillemer, K.A., & Suitor, J.J. (1992). Violence and violent feelings: What causes them among family givers? *Journal of Gerontology 47*:S165-S172.

Ramsey-Klawsnik, H. (2000). Elder-abuse offenders: A typology. *Generations, 26*(2), 17-22.

Reis, M., & Nahmiah, D. (1998). Validation of the indicators of abuse (IOA) screen. *The Gerontologist 38*(4):471-480.

United Nations Population Division: World Population Aging: 1950-2050, Retrieved December 19, 2004 from *http://www.un.org/esa/population/publications/worldageing 19502050/index.htm*

Widlack, P. A., Greenley, J. R., & McKee, D. (1992). Validity of case manager reports of clients' functioning in the community: Independent living, income, employment, family contact, and problem behaviors. *Community Mental Health Journal, 28*(6), 505-517.

Wolf, R. S. (2000). The nature and scope of elder abuse. *Generations, 14*(11), 6-12.

Wolf, R.S., & Pillemer, K. (1989). *Helping Elderly Victims: The Reality of Elder Abuse.* New York: Columbia University Press.

Wolf, R. S., Strugnell, C. P. & Godkin, M.A. (1982). *Preliminary Findings from Three Model Projects on Elderly Abuse, Center on Aging.* Worcester, MA: University of Massachusetts Medical Center.

APPENDIX A

Level of Dependency Scale

Case #_____

On a scale of 1 to 5, with 1 indicating "not at all dependent" and 5 indicating " completely dependent," in your opinion, how dependent is the ABUSER on the VICTIM for:

	Not at all				Completely	Don't Know
1. A place to live	1	2	3	4	5	8
2. Everyday expenses, such as food, clothing, transportation costs	1	2	3	4	5	8
3. Cooking and cleaning	1	2	3	4	5	8
4. Caring for their children (your grandchildren)	1	2	3	4	5	8

On a scale of 1 to 5, with 1 indicating "not at all dependent" and 5 indicating "completely dependent," in your opinion, how dependent is the VICTIM on the ABUSER for:

	Not at all				Completely	Don't Know
1. Pay rent	1	2	3	4	5	8
2. Buy food, clothing, or pay for transportation costs	1	2	3	4	5	8
3. Prepare meals	1	2	3	4	5	8
4. Clean apartment	1	2	3	4	5	8
5. To pay phone bill or heat bill, medications	1	2	3	4	5	8
6. Take medications, walk, dress, or bathe	1	2	3	4	5	8

APPENDIX B

Original Dependency Scale

Elder Abuse Survey DRAFT 1
TIME ONE

SECTION II Dependency Measure PART I

People often need help from family members. Do you need help from_____in any of the following areas? (Please circle)

(1) Do you need help from_____to pay your rent?   0. No   1. Yes

    a. If yes, does_____do this reliably?   0. Never   1. Sometimes   2. Always

(2) Do you need help from_____for living expenses?   0. No   1. Yes

    a. If yes, does_____do this reliably?   0. Never   1. Sometimes   2. Always

(3) Do you need help from_____to shop for groceries or clothes? 0. No   1. Yes

    a. If yes, does_____do this reliably?   0. Never   1. Sometimes   2. Always

(4) Do you need help from_____to prepare your meals? 0. No   1. Yes

    a. If yes, does_____do this reliably?   0. Never   1. Sometimes   2. Always

(5) Do you need help from_____to clean your apartment?   0. No   1. Yes

    a. If yes, does_____do this reliably?   0. Never   1. Sometimes   2. Always

(6) Do you need help from_____for transportation?   0. No   1. Yes

    a. If yes, does_____do this reliably?   0. Never   1. Sometimes   2. Always

(7) Do you need help from_____to take medications? 0. Yes   1. No

    a. If yes, does_____do this reliably?   0. Never   1. Sometimes   2. Always

(8) Do you need help from_____to get in and out of bed?   0. No   1. Yes
   (If no, skip to Part II)

    a. If yes, does_____do this reliably?   0. Never   1. Sometimes 2. Always

(9) Do you need help from_____to walk?   0. No 1. Yes
   (If no, please skip to part II)

    a. If yes, does_____do this reliably?   0. Never   1. Sometimes 2. Always

(10) Do you need help from_____for bathing and dressing?   0. No   1. Yes
   (if no, please skip to Part II)

    a. If yes, does_____do this reliably?   0. Never   1. Sometimes 2. Always

APPENDIX B

Part II of Section II

It is possible that_____needs help from you in certain areas. To what extent does_____depend on you in the following areas?

	Entirely Dependent	Somewhat Dependent	Independent	Unknown
1. A place to live	1	2	3	4
2. Everyday expenses	1	2	3	4
3. Cooking and cleaning	1	2	3	4
4. Food	1	2	3	4
5. Caring for their children (your grandchildren)	1	2	3	4

Index

BOOK ORDER FORM!

Order a copy of this book with this form or online at:
http://www.haworthpress.com/store/product.asp?sku= 5710

Elder Abuse and Mistreatment
Policy, Practice, and Research

____ in softbound at $29.95 ISBN-13: 978-0-7890-3023-8 / ISBN-10: 0-7890-3023-3.
____ in hardbound at $49.95 ISBN-13: 978-0-7890-3022-1 / ISBN-10: 0-7890-3022-5.

COST OF BOOKS _____

POSTAGE & HANDLING _____
US: $4.00 for first book & $1.50
for each additional book
Outside US: $5.00 for first book
& $2.00 for each additional book.

SUBTOTAL _____
In Canada: add 7% GST. _____

STATE TAX _____
CA, IL, IN, MN, NJ, NY, OH, PA & SD residents
please add appropriate local sales tax.

FINAL TOTAL _____
If paying in Canadian funds, convert
using the current exchange rate,
UNESCO coupons welcome.

❏ BILL ME LATER:
Bill-me option is good on US/Canada/
Mexico orders only; not good to jobbers,
wholesalers, or subscription agencies.

❏ Signature _____

Payment Enclosed: $ _____

❏ PLEASE CHARGE TO MY CREDIT CARD:
❏ Visa ❏ MasterCard ❏ AmEx ❏ Discover
❏ Diner's Club ❏ Eurocard ❏ JCB

Account # _____

Exp Date _____

Signature _____
(Prices in US dollars and subject to change without notice.)

PLEASE PRINT ALL INFORMATION OR ATTACH YOUR BUSINESS CARD

Name	
Address	
City	State/Province	Zip/Postal Code
Country	
Tel	Fax

May we use your e-mail address for confirmations and other types of information? ❏ Yes ❏ No We appreciate receiving
your e-mail address. Haworth would like to e-mail special discount offers to you, as a preferred customer.
We will never share, rent, or exchange your e-mail address. We regard such actions as an invasion of your privacy.

Order from your **local bookstore** or directly from
The Haworth Press, Inc. 10 Alice Street, Binghamton, New York 13904-1580 • USA
Call our toll-free number (1-800-429-6784) / Outside US/Canada: (607) 722-5857
Fax: 1-800-895-0582 / Outside US/Canada: (607) 771-0012
E-mail your order to us: orders@haworthpress.com

For orders outside US and Canada, you may wish to order through your local
sales representative, distributor, or bookseller.
For information, see http://haworthpress.com/distributors

(Discounts are available for individual orders in US and Canada only, not booksellers/distributors.)

Please photocopy this form for your personal use.
www.HaworthPress.com

BOF06